Multiple Sclerosis, Part II: Nonconventional MRI Techniques

Guest Editor

MASSIMO FILIPPI, MD

NEUROIMAGING CLINICS OF NORTH AMERICA

www.neuroimaging.theclinics.com

Consulting Editor
SURESH K. MUKHERJI, MD

February 2009 • Volume 19 • Number 1

SAUNDERS an imprint of ELSEVIER, Inc.

W.B. SAUNDERS COMPANY
A Division of Elsevier Inc.

1600 John F. Kennedy Boulevard • Suite 1800 • Philadelphia, Pennsylvania 19103-2899

http://www.theclinics.com

NEUROIMAGING CLINICS OF NORTH AMERICA Volume 19, Number 1
February 2009 ISSN 1052-5149, ISBN 13: 978-1-4377-0502-7, ISBN 10: 1-4377-0502-2

Editor: Donald Mumford

Neuroimaging Clinics of North America (ISSN 1052-5149) is published quarterly by Elsevier Inc., 360 Park Avenue South, New York, NY 10010-1710. Months of issue are February, May, August, and November. Business and editorial offices: 1600 John F. Kennedy Blvd., Suite 1800, Philadelphia, PA 19103-2899. Business and editorial offices: 6277 Sea Harbor Drive, Orlando, FL 32887-4800. Periodicals postage paid at New York, NY, and additional mailing offices. Subscription prices are USD 264 per year for US individuals, USD 407 per year for US institutions, USD 135 per year for US students and residents, USD 305 per year for Canadian individuals, USD 510 per year for Canadian institutions, USD 388 per year for international individuals, USD 510 per year for international institutions and USD 194 per year for Canadian and foreign students and residents. To receive student/resident rate, orders must be accompanied by name of affiliated institution, date of term, and the *signature* of program/residency coordinator on institution letterhead. Orders will be billed at individual rate until proof of status is received. Foreign air speed delivery is included in all *Clinics* subscription prices. All prices are subject to change without notice. POSTMASTER: Send address changes to *Neuroimaging Clinics of North America*, Elsevier Periodicals Customer Service, 11830 Westline Industrial Drive, St. Louis, MO 63146. Customer Service (orders, claims, online, change of address): Elsevier Periodicals Customer Service, 11830 Westline Industrial Drive, St. Louis, MO 63146. Tel: 1-800-654-2452 (U.S. and Canada); 314-453-7041 (outside U.S. and Canada). Fax: 314-453-5170. E-mail: journalscustomerservice-usa@elsevier.com (for print support); journalsonlinesupport-usa@elsevier.com (for online support).

Reprints. For copies of 100 or more of articles in this publication, please contact the Commercial Reprints Department, Elsevier Inc., 360 Park Avenue South, New York, NY 10010-1710. Tel.: 212-633-3812; Fax: 212-462-1935; E-mail: reprints@elsevier.com.

Neuroimaging Clinics of North America is covered by *Excerpta Medical/EMBASE,* the RSNA Index of Imaging Literature, *MEDLINE/PubMed (Index Medicus),* MEDLINE/MEDLARS, SciSearch, Research Alert, and Neuroscience Citation Index.

Printed in the United States of America.

GOAL STATEMENT

The goal of *Neuroimaging Clinics of North America* is to keep practicing radiologists and radiology residents up to date with current clinical practice in radiology by providing timely articles reviewing the state of the art in patient care.

ACCREDITATION

The *Neuroimaging Clinics of North America* is planned and implemented in accordance with the Essential Areas and Policies of the Accreditation Council for Continuing Medical Education (ACCME) through the joint sponsorship of the University of Virginia School of Medicine and Elsevier. The University of Virginia School of Medicine is accredited by the ACCME to provide continuing medical education for physicians.

The University of Virginia School of Medicine designates this educational activity for a maximum of 60 *AMA PRA Category 1 Credits*™. Physicians should only claim credit commensurate with the extent of their participation in the activity.

The American Medical Association has determined that physicians not licensed in the US who participate in this CME activity are eligible for *AMA PRA Category 1 Credits*™.

Credit can be earned by reading the text material, taking the CME examination online at http://www.theclinics.com/home/cme, and completing the evaluation. After taking the test, you will be required to review any and all incorrect answers. Following completion of the test and evaluation, your credit will be awarded and you may print your certificate.

FACULTY DISCLOSURE/CONFLICT OF INTEREST

The University of Virginia School of Medicine, as an ACCME accredited provider, endorses and strives to comply with the Accreditation Council for Continuing Medical Education (ACCME) Standards of Commercial Support, Commonwealth of Virginia statutes, University of Virginia policies and procedures, and associated federal and private regulations and guidelines on the need for disclosure and monitoring of proprietary and financial interests that may affect the scientific integrity and balance of content delivered in continuing medical education activities under our auspices.

The University of Virginia School of Medicine requires that all CME activities accredited through this institution be developed independently and be scientifically rigorous, balanced and objective in the presentation/discussion of its content, theories and practices.

All authors/editors participating in an accredited CME activity are expected to disclose to the readers relevant financial relationships with commercial entities occurring within the past 12 months (such as grants or research support, employee, consultant, stock holder, member of speakers bureau, etc.). The University of Virginia School of Medicine will employ appropriate mechanisms to resolve potential conflicts of interest to maintain the standards of fair and balanced education to the reader. Questions about specific strategies can be directed to the Office of Continuing Medical Education, University of Virginia School of Medicine, Charlottesville, Virginia.

The faculty and staff of the University of Virginia Office of Continuing Medical Education have no financial affiliations to disclose.

The authors/editors listed below have identified no professional/financial affiliations for themselves or their spouse/partner:

Federica Agosta, MD; Frederik Barkhof, MD, PhD; Joseph CJ. Bot, MD, PhD; Steven L. Galetta, MD; Christopher C. Glisson, DO, MS; Alayar Kangarlu, PhD; Shannon H. Kolind, MSc; Cornelia Laule, PhD; Alex L. MacKay, DPhil; Elisabetta Pagani, PhD; Alexander Rauscher, PhD; Lisa Richman (Acquiring Editor); Maria Assunta Rocca, MD; Stefan Ropele, PhD; Marco Rovaris, MD; Balasrinivasa R. Sajja, PhD; and Irene M. Vavasour, PhD.

The authors listed below have identified the following professional/financial affiliations for themselves or their spouse/partner:

Franz Fazekas, MD is an industry funded research/investigator, consultant, serves on the Speakers Bureau and Advisory Committee for Biogen Idec, Bayer Schering, Merck Serono, and Teva/Sanofi Aventis.

Massimo Filippi, MD (Guest Editor) is an industry funded research/investigator, consultant, and serves on the Speakers Bureau for TEVA Pharmaceutical Industries, Merck-Serono, Bayer-Schering, and Biogen Dompe.

David K. B. Li, MD is the director of the UBC MS/MRI Research Group that has performed trials with Angiotech, Bayer, Berlex-Schering, BioMS, Centocor, Daiichi Sankyo, Hoffmann-LaRoche, Merck-Serono, Schering-Plough, Teva Neurosciences, Sanofi-Aventis, and Transition Therapeutics.

Burkard Mädler, PhD is employed by Philips Healthcare.

Paul M. Matthews, DPhil, FRCP is employed by and owns stock in GlaxoSmithKline.

G.R. Wayne Moore, MD is a consultant and an industry funded research/investigator for Bayer.

Suresh K. Mukherji, MD (Consulting Editor) is a consultant for Bracco, Bayer, Philips, and Xoran Technologies.

Ponnada A. Narayana, PhD is a sponsor of a workshop with Teva Neuroscience.

Anthony L. Traboulsee, MD serves on the Speakers Bureau for EMD Serono and Teva Neurosciences.

Jerry S. Wolinsky, MD is a consultant for AstraZeneca, EMD Serono, and Glycominds, is a consultant and serves on the Advisory Committee for Teva Pharmaceuticals, Teva Neurosciences, Genentech, Inc., sanofi-aventis, and Novartis, serves on the Speakers Bureau for WebMD Corp., and BCDecker, serves on the Advisory Committee for Protein Deign Labs, Bayer (Schering), European Charcot Foundation and BioPartners, Antisense Therapeutics, Ltd., and UCB, has received grants from National Institutes of Health and Clayton Foundation for Research, and is an industry funded research/investigator for Sanofi-Aventis.

Disclosure of Discussion of Non-FDA Approved Uses for Pharmaceutical Products and/or Medical Devices.

The University of Virginia School of Medicine, as an ACCME provider, requires that all faculty presenters identify and disclose any off-label uses for pharmaceutical and medical device products. The University of Virginia School of Medicine recommends that each physician fully review all the available data on new products or procedures prior to clinical use.

TO ENROLL

To enroll in the Neuroimaging Clinics of North America Continuing Medical Education program, call customer service at 1-800-654-2452 or sign up online at *http://www.theclinics.com/home/cme*. The CME program is available to subscribers for an additional annual fee of USD 175.

Neuroimaging Clinics of North America

THE CLINICS ARE NOW AVAILABLE ONLINE!

Access your subscription at:
www.theclinics.com

Contributors

CONSULTING EDITOR

SURESH K. MUKHERJI, MD
Professor and Chief of Neuroradiology and
Head and Neck Radiology; Professor of
Radiology, Otolaryngology Head Neck Surgery
and Radiation Oncology, University of
Michigan Health System, Ann Arbor, Michigan

GUEST EDITOR

MASSIMO FILIPPI, MD
Director, Neuroimaging Research Unit,
Department of Neurology, San Raffaele
Scientific Institute and University, Milan, Italy

AUTHORS

FEDERICA AGOSTA, MD
Neuroimaging Research Unit, Department
of Neurology, San Raffaele Scientific Institute
and University, Milan, Italy

FREDERIK BARKHOF, MD, PhD
Department of Radiology, MR Center for MS
Research, VU Medical Center, Amsterdam,
The Netherlands

JOSEPH CJ. BOT, MD, PhD
Department of Radiology, MR Center for MS
Research, VU Medical Center, Amsterdam,
The Netherlands

FRANZ FAZEKAS, MD
Department of Neurology, Medical University
Graz, Austria

MASSIMO FILIPPI, MD
Director, Neuroimaging Research Unit,
Department of Neurology, San Raffaele
Scientific Institute and University, Milan, Italy

STEVEN L. GALETTA, MD
Director of Neuro-Ophthalmology, Division
of Neuro-Ophthalmology, Department
of Neurology, University of Pennsylvania
School of Medicine; Director of
Neuro-Ophthalmology, Division of
Neuro-Ophthalmology, Department
of Ophthalmology, University of Pennsylvania
School of Medicine, Philadelphia,
Pennsylvania

CHRISTOPHER C. GLISSON, DO, MS
Department of Neurology and Ophthalmology,
Michigan State University College of Human
Medicine; Medical Director of
Neuro-Ophthalmology, Saint Mary's Health
Care, Grand Rapids, Michigan

ALAYAR KANGARLU, PhD
Columbia University College of Physicians and
Surgeons and New York State Psychiatric
Institute, New York, New York

S.H. KOLIND, MSc
Department of Physics and Astronomy, University of British Columbia; UBC MRI Research Centre, Department of Radiology, UBC Hospital, Vancouver, British Columbia, Canada

C. LAULE, PhD
Department of Radiology, University of British Columbia; UBC MRI Research Centre, Department of Radiology, UBC Hospital, Vancouver, British Columbia, Canada

D.K.B. LI, MD
Department of Radiology, University of British Columbia; UBC MRI Research Centre, Department of Radiology, UBC Hospital, Vancouver, British Columbia, Canada

A.L. MᴀᴄKAY, DPhil
Department of Radiology, University of British Columbia; Department of Physics and Astronomy, University of British Columbia; UBC MRI Research Centre, Department of Radiology, UBC Hospital, Vancouver, British Columbia, Canada

B. MÄDLER, PhD
UBC MRI Research Centre, Department of Radiology, UBC Hospital, Canada; Philips Healthcare, Vancouver, British Columbia, Canada

PAUL M. MATTHEWS, DPhil, FRCP
Head and Vice President for Imaging, Glaxo Smith Kline Clinical Imaging Centre, Hammersmith Hospital; Professor of Clinical Neurosciences, Department of Clinical Neurosciences, Imperial College, London, United Kingdom

G.R.W. MOORE, MD
UBC MRI Research Centre, Department of Radiology, UBC Hospital; Department of Pathology and Laboratory Medicine, University of British Columbia, Vancouver, British Columbia, Canada

PONNADA A. NARAYANA, PhD
Department of Diagnostic and Interventional Imaging, University of Texas Medical School at Houston, Houston, Texas

ELISABETTA PAGANI, PhD
Neuroimaging Research Unit, Department of Neurology, San Raffaele Scientific Institute and University, Milan, Italy

A. RAUSCHER, PhD
Department of Radiology, University of British Columbia; UBC MRI Research Centre, Department of Radiology, UBC Hospital, Vancouver, British Columbia, Canada

M.A. ROCCA, MD
Neuroimaging Research Unit, Department of Neurology, San Raffaele Scientific Institute and University, Milan, Italy

STEFAN ROPELE, PhD
Department of Neurology, Medical University Graz, Austria

MARCO ROVARIS, MD
Neuroimaging Research Unit, Department of Neurology, San Raffaele Scientific Institute and University; Multiple Sclerosis Unit, Scientific Institute Santa Maria Nascente—Fondazione Don Gnocchi, Milan, Italy

BALASRINIVASA R. SAJJA, PhD
Department of Radiology, University of Nebraska Medical Center, Nebraska Medical Center, Omaha, Nebraska

A.L. TRABOULSEE, MD
UBC MRI Research Centre, Department of Radiology, UBC Hospital; Department of Medicine, University of British Columbia, Vancouver, British Columbia, Canada

I.M. VAVASOUR, PhD
Department of Radiology, University of British Columbia; UBC MRI Research Centre, Department of Radiology, UBC Hospital, Vancouver, British Columbia, Canada

JERRY S. WOLINSKY, MD
Department of Neurology, University of Texas Medical School at Houston, Houston, Texas

Contents

> This article provides an overview of relaxation times and their application to normal brain and brain and cord affected by multiple sclerosis. The goal is to provide readers with an intuitive understanding of what influences relaxation times, how relaxation times can be accurately measured, and how they provide specific information about the pathology of MS. The article summarizes significant results from relaxation time studies in the normal human brain and cord and from people who have multiple sclerosis. It also reports on studies that have compared relaxation time results with results from other MR techniques.

> We introduce the fundamental aspects of MT, of MT MR imaging, and the respective analysis techniques. We then review the applications of MT MR imaging to multiple sclerosis. Finally we review the technique's contribution to our understanding of this disease.

> Diffusion tensor (DT) MR imaging is able to detect and quantify multiple sclerosis (MS)–related tissue damage within and outside T2-visible lesions. DT MR imaging has also been shown to be sensitive to the evolution of MS damage over time and to provide in vivo correlates of MS clinical severity and paraclinical markers of long-term disease evolution. Recent developments of DT MR imaging postprocessing techniques, such as tractography and voxelwise analysis, are likely to improve our understanding of the mechanisms associated with the accumulation of disability in MS. Important issues remain to be addressed, such as a detailed definition of the actual features underlying diffusion changes in MS and the potential of the technique in the differential diagnosis of MS.

Proton magnetic resonance spectroscopy (^{1}H-MRS) provides tissue metabolic information in vivo. This article reviews the role of MRS-determined metabolic alterations in lesions, normal-appearing white matter, gray matter, and spinal cord in advancing our knowledge of pathologic changes in multiple sclerosis (MS). In addition, the role of MRS in objectively evaluating therapeutic efficacy is reviewed. This potential metabolic information makes MRS a unique tool to follow MS disease evolution, understand its pathogenesis, evaluate the disease severity, establish a prognosis, and objectively evaluate the efficacy of therapeutic interventions.

A variable effectiveness of reparative and recovery mechanisms following tissue damage is among the factors that might contribute to explaining resolution of symptoms and maintenance of a normal level of function in patients who have multiple sclerosis (MS). The application of functional MR imaging in MS has shown that cortical changes do occur after white matter injury and that these changes can contribute to limiting the clinical outcome of such damage. Conversely, the failure or exhaustion of the adaptive properties of the cerebral cortex with increasing disease duration and burden might be among the factors responsible for the accumulation of fixed neurologic deficits in patients who have MS.

Conventional MR imaging is, at present, the most important paraclinical modality for assessing the risk of MS in patients with acute demyelinating ON and for monitoring the progression of disease. However, there are limitations of conventional MR in imaging the optic nerve. Newer strategies, MT MR imaging, DT MR imaging, and OCT, show significant promise. Future investigations, including the use of nonconventional MR imaging techniques coupled with OCT and functional measures of anterior visual pathway function, will further assist in the early detection of clinical impairment. Serial analysis will allow for monitoring of disease progression, predict accumulation of disability, and ascertain the effects of candidate neuroprotective therapies.

Multiple sclerosis is a diffuse disease of the central nervous system, and MRI of the spinal cord is highly recommended in the clinical evaluation of patients suspected of having multiple sclerosis. Within the new diagnostic criteria, spinal cord MRI increases sensitivity and possibly specificity for MS, but further work is needed to investigate other criteria that may give greater weight to the presence of cord lesions in patients with clinically isolated syndromes or suspected relapsing-remitting multiple sclerosis. Techniques should be further studied and validated in studies comparing these techniques with clinical status and histopathology, however.

Brain Imaging of Multiple Sclerosis: the Next 10 Years   101
Paul M. Matthews

MR imaging has had a major impact on understanding the dynamic neuropathologic findings of multiple sclerosis (MS), early diagnosis of the disease, and clinical trial conduct. The next 10 years can be expected to see further advances with a greater emphasis on large multicenter studies, new techniques and hardware allowing greater imaging sensitivity and resolution, and the exploitation of positron emission tomography molecular imaging for MS. The impact should be felt with a new emphasis on gray matter disease and processes of repair. With new ways of monitoring the disease, new treatment targets should become practical, helping to translate advances in the understanding of immunology and regenerative medicine into novel therapies.

High-Field Magnetic Resonance Imaging   113
Alayar Kangarlu

This article explores the role of high-field (HF) MR imaging in medicine. It analyzes advantages of HF MR imaging in application to human subjects and how best they can be used to unravel the secrets of diseases, such as multiple sclerosis. Special emphasis is placed on morphologic imaging to highlight the role of soft tissue contrast, MR spectroscopy to showcase the ability of detecting biochemical information, and functional MR imaging as an emerging technology for assessing tissue function with the possibility of eventual introduction to the clinical arena. In this article, hardware issues, such as RF coils for HF systems with a static magnetic field of 3.0 T or higher are also discussed.

Foreword

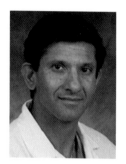

Suresh K. Mukherji, MD
Consulting Editor

Once again, we are very honored to have Dr. Massimo Filippi as our Guest Editor for *Neuroimaging Clinics of North America*. Dr. Filippi is a recognized expert in multiple sclerosis (MS), and his numerous contributions are known throughout the world. He is Director of the Neuroimaging Research Unit in the Department of Neurology at the San Raffaele Scientific Institute and University in Milan, Italy. He also has academic affiliations at Temple University and the University of Belgrade.

Dr. Filippi's contribution to *Neuroimaging Clinics of North America* has been comprised of two issues. This two-part series is a dedicated translational treatise covering all aspects of MS. The first issue was entitled "Background and Conventional MRI" and reviewed the pathology, epidemiology, immunology, and clinical manifestations of MS. This information is necessary for understanding this complex disease and forms the foundation for subsequent articles on the imaging findings. This second issue focuses on the most promising MRI techniques under development or that have recently emerged and are likely to have a substantial impact on the treatment and management of MS. These techniques include magnetization transfer, diffusion tensor imaging, fMRI, and MR spectroscopy.

I would like to personally thank Dr. Filippi for his tireless efforts in the preparation of this work, as well as the numerous authors for their wonderful contributions. The list of authors is literally a who's-who of internationally recognized investigators and thought leaders in MS.

MR appears to be an optimal modality to investigate MS, as the physiologic applications of MR imaging can be used to evaluate different aspects of MS pathology. From Dr. Filippi's contribution, it is clear that combined information available from MR imaging can be used for both diagnosis and treatment monitoring. This information can also be used to further increase our understanding of the underlying disease mechanisms and possibly predict the accumulation of disability. All of us in the scientific community sincerely thank Dr. Filippi and the contributing authors for their unprecedented contribution to *Neuroimaging Clinics of North America*. It is our hope that this important material will benefit all individuals whose lives have been touched by MS. This includes clinicians, investigators, and, most importantly, our patients.

Suresh K. Mukherji, MD
Neuroradiology and Head and Neck Radiology
Radiology, Otolaryngology Head Neck Surgery
and Radiation Oncology
University of Michigan Health System
1500 E. Medical Center Drive
Ann Arbor, MI 48109-0030, USA

E-mail address:
mukherji@med.umich.edu (S.K. Mukherji)

Neuroimag Clin N Am 19 (2009) xi
doi:10.1016/j.nic.2008.10.002
1052-5149/08/$ – see front matter © 2008 Elsevier Inc. All rights reserved.

Preface

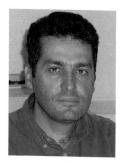

Massimo Filippi, MD
Guest Editor

This is the second issue of *Neuroimaging Clinics of North America* dealing with the application of magnetic resonance imaging (MRI) in multiple sclerosis (MS). It aims to provide an overview of the technical and clinical issues related to the role of modern, quantitative MRI techniques in the understanding of this disease. The first part was devoted to the main pathological, epidemiological, immunological, and clinical aspects of MS and provided the background of basic principles of MR and the strategies more commonly used for data analysis. The first issue also offered an overview of how conventional MRI is applied in the monitoring of disease evolution, both natural or modified by treatment.

This second issue considers the most promising MRI approaches to the study of MS that have emerged recently or are under development/ refinement and are likely to impact significantly the clinical arena in the near future. Indeed, these techniques have undoubtedly contributed to define the mechanisms through which MS causes the accumulation of irreversible disability. For instance, their application to MS has shown that the pathology of the disease is not limited to macroscopic focal lesions but also involves diffusely the normal-appearing white (NAWM) and gray matter (GM), directly or through retrograde and transsynaptic degeneration. Correlative pathological/MRI studies have also demonstrated that these MRI techniques may have a different sensitivity towards the heterogeneous pathological substrates of the disease (which, among the many others, include axonal loss, demyelination, and remyelination), and, as a consequence, might provide a valuable tool for their in vivo monitoring. The majority of the techniques that are discussed

here provide quantitative, objective, and reproducible measures of disease severity that are likely to improve the strength of the correlation between clinical and MRI findings in MS. It is foreseen that, if adequately optimized and standardized across centers, they might be applied in the near future in clinical trials to monitor tissue damage and repair.

The first section of this issue describes the main results and reports critically the advantages and pitfalls obtained from the clinical use of such modern MR techniques. The first article focuses on relaxation time measurements, which, albeit not popular yet, can provide specific and accurate pieces of information on MS pathology. The application of relaxation time measurements to both normal and MS brain and spinal cord is discussed in order to provide the reader with an understanding of the matter. A comparison of the results obtained with relaxation time measurements and those from other MR techniques, such as diffusion tensor (DT) and magnetization transfer (MT) MRI, is also given. These latter two techniques are discussed, separately and extensively, in the subsequent two articles, which show how much we have learned from their use in the last decade or so. Due to its unique advantage to provide information with high biochemical specificity for tissue changes, proton magnetic resonance spectroscopy (^{1}H-MRS) is then reviewed. Among the many ^{1}H-MRS-derived metabolic measures, the level of N-acetylaspartate (NAA) represents a highly specific correlate of neuronal and axonal viability.

Despite the sensitivity of relaxation time measurements, MT MRI, DT MRI, and ^{1}H-MRS to disease changes, the correlation between quantitative MR-derived measures of tissue integrity

Neuroimag Clin N Am 19 (2009) xiii–xiv
doi:10.1016/j.nic.2008.10.001

neuroimaging.theclinics.com

and clinical scales of impairment/disability are still scanty. During the last few years, the availability and then the extensive application of functional MRI to the assessment of central nervous system (CNS) function in MS patients has demonstrated that the presence and efficacy of brain adaptive mechanisms might contribute, at least in some phases of the disease, to limiting clinical consequences of diffuse disease-related tissue injury and, conversely, that the failure of such mechanisms might be among the factors responsible for the accumulation of irreversible disability. All these aspects are discussed in the article devoted to this technique. The last two papers of this section review the studies that applied quantitative MRI techniques to the assessment of structure and function of the optic nerve and spinal cord, two eloquent CNS regions that are frequently involved by the disease and, due to their characteristics, might serve as a model to improve our understanding of MS. Technical advancement that has occurred during the last decade has allowed a more precise quantification of tissue integrity of the optic nerve and spinal cord and, as a consequence, it is likely to result in a better definition of the picture of the disease.

The unprecedented and extensive evolution of conventional and quantitative MR-based techniques and their application to the study of MS has undoubtedly improved our ability to diagnose and monitor the disease, as well as our understanding of its pathophysiology. Nevertheless, there are many remaining challenges in front of us. New techniques need to be refined and validated before they can be integrated properly into clinical research and practice. New acquisition schemes and analysis procedures require standardization and optimization so that they can be used in multi-site settings. From the data presently available, it is becoming clear that combining different MR modalities, which are sensitive to different aspects of MS pathology, is a promising way to increase further our understanding of the mechanisms accounting for the accumulation of disability. Finally, the increasing availability of high-field strength MRI (3.0 T and higher) presents a new set of challenges that require extensive refinement during the next few years. All of these aspects are discussed in the last two contributions to this issue, which also aims to delineate a map of future research over the next ten years.

Massimo Filippi, MD
Neuroimaging Research Unit
Department of Neurology
San Raffaele Scientific Institute and University
Via Olgettina, 60-20132, Milan, Italy

E-mail address:
filippi.massimo@hsr.it (M. Filippi)

MR Relaxation in Multiple Sclerosis

A.L. MacKay, DPhil[a,b,c,*], I.M. Vavasour, PhD[a,c], A. Rauscher, PhD[a,c],
S.H. Kolind, MSc[b,c], B. Mädler, PhD[c,d], G.R.W. Moore, MD[c,e],
A.L. Traboulsee, MD[c,f], D.K.B. Li, MD[a,c], C. Laule, PhD[a,c]

KEYWORDS

- Relaxation • T_1 • T_2 • Brain • Multiple sclerosis

OVERVIEW

Relaxation is arguably the most important concept in MRI because it is the basis of and provides most of the contrast visible on conventional MRI, which plays a key role in the diagnosis and management of multiple sclerosis (MS). Many investigators have attempted to measure relaxation times in MS with the goal of obtaining more specific and accurate information about the disease. Although there has been significant progress in this area, relaxation time measurement is not yet a widely used tool for the investigation of MS pathology. Recent results suggest that relaxation time measurements can provide specific information about MS that cannot be obtained by other in vivo techniques.

This article provides an overview of relaxation times and their application to normal and MS brain and cord. The goal is to provide readers with an intuitive understanding of what influences relaxation times, how relaxation times can be accurately measured, and how they provide specific information about the pathology of MS. The article is organized into six sections. First, three relaxation times—T1, T2, and T2*—are introduced, initially in the context of their behavior in simple water solutions and subsequently in central nervous system (CNS) tissue, where MR relaxation is much

more complicated. The next section covers methods for accurate measurement and analysis of relaxation times in brain, highlighting the fact that CNS tissue is inhomogeneous and that this inhomogeneity can be planned for in the methodology. The article summarizes significant results from relaxation time studies in the normal human brain and cord and from people who have MS. Finally the article reports on studies that have compared relaxation time results with results from other MR techniques, including diffusion tensor imaging (DTI) and magnetization transfer imaging.

Although this article focuses primarily on T1, T2, and T2* relaxation times, susceptibility-weighted imaging (SWI), a T2* weighted technique is discussed. This article does not cover all relaxation time measurements (eg, T1ρ and T2ρ) because few MS studies have used these measurements.

T1, T2, AND T2* RELAXATION TIMES
Nuclear Magnetic Resonance

The phenomenon of nuclear magnetic resonance (NMR) enables us to obtain exquisite images from hydrogen nuclei in the brain. Hydrogen nuclei, or protons, from tissue behave like tiny magnets when placed in the magnetic field of an MRI scanner. In equilibrium, more protons are aligned

This work was supported by the Multiple Sclerosis Society of Canada and the Natural Sciences and Engineering Research Council.
[a] Department of Radiology, University of British Columbia, Vancouver, BC, Canada
[b] Department of Physics and Astronomy, University of British Columbia, Vancouver, BC, Canada
[c] UBC MRI Research Centre, Department of Radiology, Room M10, Purdy Pavilion, UBC Hospital, 2221 Wesbrook Mall, Vancouver BC V6T 2B5 Canada
[d] Philips Healthcare, Vancouver BC Canada
[e] Department of Pathology and Laboratory Medicine, University of British Columbia, Vancouver, BC, Canada
[f] Department of Medicine, University of British Columbia, Vancouver, BC, Canada
* Corresponding author. UBC MRI Research Centre, Department of Radiology, Room M10, Purdy Pavilion, UBC Hospital, 2221 Wesbrook Mall, Vancouver BC V6T 2B5 Canada.
E-mail address: mackay@physics.ubc.ca (A. MacKay).

Neuroimag Clin N Am 19 (2009) 1–26
doi:10.1016/j.nic.2008.09.007
1052-5149/08/$ – see front matter

parallel to the field than anti-parallel to the field, which results in a net magnetization vector along the magnetic field. If the net magnetization vector of the protons is tilted away from the MRI scanner field direction, it precesses about the direction of the magnetic field (like a top or gyroscope) at the resonance frequency, or Larmor frequency, ω_o. ω_o, which is determined by the Larmor equation, $\omega_o = \gamma B$, where γ, the gyromagnetic ratio, depends on the nucleus and B is the magnetic field. For a 1.5-T magnet, the Larmor frequency for protons is 64 MHz. The magnetization vector is tilted out of equilibrium by applying external magnetic fields that oscillate at the Larmor frequency. The precessing magnetization produces a signal that can be picked up by a receiver coil and is used to create the MR image. The return of the net magnetization vector of the protons back to equilibrium is characterized by relaxation times T1, T2, and T2*.

Relaxation Times

T1, the spin–lattice relaxation time (or longitudinal relaxation time), characterizes the return of the magnetization vector to align along the magnetic field direction. T2, the spin–spin relaxation time (or transverse relaxation time), describes the irreversible decay of the MR signal in the transverse plane, whereas T2* characterizes the actual measured decay of the MR signal. The T1 process involves an exchange of energy between the protons and the rest of the sample, or lattice, whereas T2 processes conserve energy. The next section provides a mechanistic description of T1 and T2 processes; readers who prefer a more intuitive picture of relaxation in tissue may skip to the following section.

T1 and T2 Processes

For a simple spin system consisting of a molecule with a single proton site, T1 and T2 are understood quantitatively in terms of fluctuating magnetic fields produced by adjacent protons undergoing molecular motions.[1,2] Recall that protons behave like small magnets. When protons are located on molecules that reorient rapidly because of molecular tumbling and translational diffusion, they produce oscillating magnetic fields. Molecular motions, which are driven by the inherent kinetic energy of the molecules, are characterized by a correlation time, τ_c, the time required for the molecule to undergo reorientation. The fluctuating magnetic fields caused by these molecular motions cause relaxation. The dependence of T1 and T2 on the correlation time of molecular motions and Larmor frequency is quantitatively expressed in equations 1 and 2. The constant, K, is related to the strength of the interactions between adjacent protons.

$$\frac{1}{T_1} = K\left(\frac{\tau_c}{1+(\omega_o\tau_c)^2} + \frac{4\tau_c}{1+(2\omega_o\tau_c)^2}\right) \quad (1)$$

$$\frac{1}{T_2} = K\left(\frac{3}{2}\tau_c + \frac{5/2\tau_c}{1+(\omega_o\tau_c)^2} + \frac{\tau_c}{1+(2\omega_o\tau_c)^2}\right) \quad (2)$$

Equations 1 and 2 show that T1 and T2 are sensitive to rapid molecular motions at the Larmor frequency and twice the Larmor frequency. The additional term on the left of Equation 2, $3/2\ \tau_c$, is large for low-frequency motions, which explains why T2 is more sensitive than T1 to slow motions. **Fig. 1** plots T1 and T2 using equations 1 and 2 at 1.5 T for a simple single spin system, like protons in a water solution, as a function of the ratio of the frequency of the fluctuating field to the Larmor

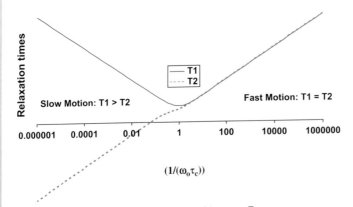

Fig. 1. Plot of relaxation times T1 and T2 as a function of the ratio of the frequency of fluctuations producing the relaxation to the Larmor frequency for 1.5 T.

frequency ($1/[\omega_o \tau_c]$). This simple model provides intuition about T1 and T2. For fast motions such as water tumbling, T1 = T2, which holds for relaxation in cerebrospinal fluid (CSF). In the presence of slow fluctuations below the Larmor frequency (64 MHz at 1.5 T), T2 is shorter than T1. For higher field MR measurements (eg, 3.0 T or 7.0 T), the Larmor frequency increases and the curves in **Fig. 1** shift upwards; this explains why T1 times increase with increasing magnetic field.

The simple model for relaxation described previously holds for simple spin systems such as water solutions but is unable to quantitatively characterize relaxation in brain that has multiple proton environments. Although the largest molecular component of brain is water (70%–80% by weight),[3] the CNS is not a simple solution but rather consists of a complex arrangement of microscopic cellular structures. In brain, there are many different proton sites. Protons attached to macromolecules and lipids do not contribute directly to the signal we measure in MRI because their signal decays to zero in a few tens of seconds.[4–6] The signal from protons attached to water in CNS tissue decays much more slowly and is fully accessible by MRI.[4,5,7,8] Relaxation times for water in CNS tissue are strongly influenced by interactions between water and nonaqueous protons, however. In pure water, relaxation is well described by a simple process with a correlation time, τ_c, of approximately 10^{-12} seconds corresponding to the fast motion regime in which T1 = T2. In brain, water protons interact with other protons attached to molecules that move at a wide range of different frequencies (eg, low frequencies that arise from slow macromolecular reorientations to high frequencies that arise from fast small molecule tumbling). As a consequence, T2 times are shorter than T1 times in CNS tissue. T1 and T2 are also shortened in the presence of indigenous ions (eg, iron from hemoglobin or ferritin), which produce fluctuating magnetic fields at high frequencies.[9,10]

Intuitive Picture of T1 and T2 in Brain

At 1.5 T, the T1 and T2 times for pure water are approximately 3 seconds, whereas the T1 time of water in brain is approximately 1 second and T2 times of water in brain are a few tens of milliseconds. This shortening in water relaxation times in CNS tissue is caused by interactions between brain water and nonaqueous tissue components, such as membranes and cytoplasmic proteins. Relaxation in brain is further complicated by the fact that local microscopic structures vary substantially within a typical imaging voxel volume of a few mm³. For example, glial cells have single plasma membranes, whereas myelinated neurons contain many membranes in close proximity. This microscopic heterogeneity results in substantially different relaxation behavior for water protons in different environments within a single voxel. As a further complication, boundaries between water environments in CNS tissue are blurred because of translational diffusion. Water molecules in pure water or dilute solutions undergo random motion, moving an average distance of $R = (6D\tau)^{1/2}$ in time τ,[11] where D is the water diffusion coefficient. For a typical MR image obtained with an echo time (TE) of 60 milliseconds, free water in a solution moves over 30 μ. The barriers present in CNS tissue suppress water diffusion coefficients to less than one tenth that in free water, and water molecules move on average 5 μ in 60 milliseconds. Because of diffusion, parameters derived by MR are averaged over their values during the timescale of the measurement. Because T2 and T1 operate on different timescales (approximately 10 milliseconds to approximately 1 second), we observe different averages with these two parameters.

Manipulating T1 and T2 Times with Exogenous Contrast Agents

Exogenous contrast agents are used to investigate blood-brain barrier breakdown in MS. Gadolinium (Gd)-based contrast agents consist of Gd ions chelated by an organic molecule that protects the body from toxic effects of the free Gd ion. When the blood-brain barrier is sufficiently leaky, chelated Gd complexes can diffuse across the vascular wall, although animal studies present some evidence that there may be active transport of Gd.[12] Water protons in the parenchyma are then exposed to intense fluctuating magnetic fields from the Gd ions. These additional high-frequency fluctuating fields cause a decrease in T1 and T2. This effect enables identification of regions of blood-brain barrier breakdown in MS brain that characterize enhancing lesions.[13] By measuring changes in signal intensity in rapidly acquired brain images after injection of a bolus of Gd contrast into the venous system, it is possible to measure brain perfusion.[14]

T2*and Susceptibility-Weighted Imaging

Magnetic susceptibility is a concept that describes a substance's ability to modify an applied magnetic field. The magnetic susceptibility, χ, is a constant that relates to the magnetization (M) of a substance by

$$\mathbf{M} = \chi \mathbf{H} \tag{3}$$

with the external magnetic field **H**. This magnetization (**M**) shifts the actual magnetic field B from **H** as shown in equation 4, where $\mu_0 = 4\pi$ $10^{-7} VsA^{-1}m^{-1}$ denotes the permeability in a vacuum.

$$B = \mu_0(H+M) \qquad (4)$$

Depending on the sign of χ, materials are referred to as diamagnetic ($\chi < 0$) or paramagnetic ($\chi > 0$). Most tissues are diamagnetic (slightly repelled by a magnetic field).[15,16] The main source of paramagnetism (form of magnetism that occurs only in the presence of an externally applied magnetic field) in the human body is iron.[15,17,18] If a sample contains two or more compartments with different magnetic susceptibilities, static magnetic field inhomogeneities arise, which fall into two categories:[19] (1) mesoscopic field inhomogeneities, which are field variations over distances longer than the water diffusion length during TE of an MR measurement but smaller than the voxel size, and (2) macroscopic field inhomogeneities, which vary over several voxels. In the human body, interfaces between air and tissue, bone and tissue, or veins and surrounding tissue are the main sources of field inhomogeneities. These inhomogeneities lead to an additional signal decay that is commonly characterized by a decay time of $1/T2'$. The decay due to both T2 and T2' relaxation is called T2* relaxation and obeys the simple equation

$$\frac{1}{T_2^*} = \frac{1}{T_2} + \frac{1}{T_2'} \qquad (5)$$

Equation 5 suggests that T2' decay is exponential, but this is only true if the resonance frequency distribution caused by the static field inhomogeneities is Lorentzian (eg, for a large number of magnetic dipoles within a voxel).[20,21] In general, T2' is not monoexponential and not exponential at all. For a small number of dipoles,[20] a vascular network,[19] or macroscopic background field inhomogeneities[22] the decay becomes nonexponential. In the presence of a single large blood vessel,[23–26] the concept of an exponential decay also fails because the geometric relationship between field inhomogeneities and the voxel geometry (spatial resolution, slice orientation, imaging point spread function) plays an important role in signal formation.[27–29] Venous vessels produce local field inhomogeneities,[25] which depend on the venous blood oxygenation and the vessel's orientation. For example, for a vessel parallel to the magnetic field, there are two discrete field strengths inside and outside of the vessel. Consequently, the spins inside and outside of the vessel have two discrete resonance frequencies that, when superimposed, lead to a distinct beat in the signal (**Fig. 2**).[23]

The blood oxygenation level dependency (BOLD) of the T2*-weighted signal that is the basis of functional MRI[30] and BOLD MR venography,[29,31] currently called SWI,[32] allows for the visualization of small venous vessels using deoxygenated venous blood as an intrinsic contrast agent.

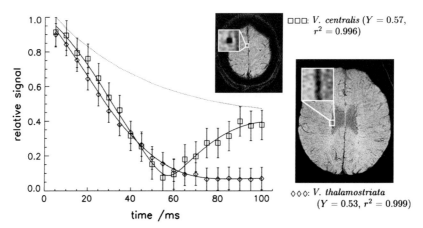

Fig. 2. The measured (*symbols*) and simulated (*solid line*) T2* signal for two veins (V. centralis, parallel to the magnetic field; V. thalamostriata, perpendicular to the magnetic field) for a healthy volunteer displays the nonexponential signal behavior caused by static field inhomogeneities. This signal formation is the basis for blood oxygen level–dependent MR venography. For the parallel vein signal recovery at late TE and a local minimum at TE approximately 55 milliseconds occur. Blood oxygenations of 0.57 and 0.53 were determined from the signal behavior. The dotted line is the signal of a homogeneous region of interest near the evaluated voxel. (*From* Sedlacik J, Rauscher A, Reichenbach JR. Obtaining blood oxygenation levels from MR signal behavior in the presence of single venous vessels. Magn Reson Med 2007;58:1035–44; with permission.)

MEASUREMENT, ANALYSIS, AND PROCESSING OF RELAXATION TIMES
Measurement of T1 Relaxation

The conventional technique for measuring T1 in vivo is the inversion recovery (IR) sequence (ie, a 180° inversion pulse followed by a variable inversion time [TI] and conventional spin echo).[1] The IR experiment provides data for a plot of MR signal as a function of TI. An example of the IR experiment and resulting T1 decay is shown in **Fig. 3**. The conventional IR sequence can be time consuming if many TI delays are required. It can be sped up considerably by replacing the spin echo with either an echo planar imaging sequence or a short repetition time (TR) gradient echo imaging sequence. A variant of the IR pulse sequence is the saturation recovery method that is a conventional spin echo sequence acquired at a series of different TRs. Another approach to measuring T1, introduced by Look and Locker,[33] involves following the 180° inversion pulse with a series of low flip angle pulses that sample the magnetization at various TI times after the initial pulse. To obtain accurate T1 estimates, it is important that the pulse sequence use sufficient TI times to sample the magnetization across the full range of signal change.

Measurement of T2 Relaxation

The Carr-Purcell-Meiboom-Gill sequence,[34,35] which consists of a 90° excitation pulse followed by a series of equally spaced 180° refocusing pulses, is the most common technique for measuring T2 times in vivo. It provides data for a plot of MR signal as a function of TE—the T2 decay curve. **Fig. 4** shows examples of T2 decay curves for pure water, normal white matter (NWM) and normal gray matter (GM), and an MS lesion. Whereas T1 times estimated from different pulse sequences should be the same, estimated T2 times may depend on the echo spacing of the multi-echo

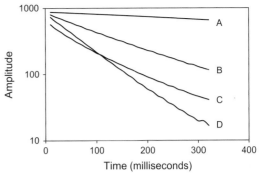

Fig. 4. Semi-logarithmic plot of T2 decay curves from pure water (A), MS lesion (B), white matter (C), and gray matter (D). Except for pure water, T2 decay curves are not mono-exponential because of multiple water compartments and require nonlinear curve fitting procedures for analysis.

sequence. The echo spacing dependence of T2 happens in the presence of effects that occur on the timescale of the interval between the 180° refocusing pulses, for example, diffusion of water between regions of different magnetic susceptibility.[9,36] Producing accurate T2 decay curves in brain in vivo is challenging because it requires accurate refocusing pulses in the presence of magnetic field and radiofrequency field inhomogeneities. An effective solution is to apply composite rectangular radiofrequency refocusing pulses flanked by large gradient pulses, which alternate in sign and decrease in height with TE.[37] The gradient pulses are required to eliminate contribution to the signal from outside the selected slice and stimulated echoes. The Poon-Henkelman multi-echo pulse sequence produces high-fidelity T2 decay curves in vivo,[7] but unfortunately it is time consuming and restricted to measuring a single slice. This two-dimensional, multi-echo, single-slice pulse sequence cannot be simply extended to a multi-slice acquisition because various microscopic environments in brain are affected differently by magnetization transfer (MT) caused by the off resonant slice selective refocusing pulses from neighboring slices.[38]

Recently, significant progress was made in speeding up the acquisition of T2 decay curves from brain. Oh and colleagues[39] implemented a novel spiral acquisition technique[40] that collected images at 12 TE times for 16 10-mm slices in 10 minutes. Mädler and MacKay[41] developed a three-dimensional multi-echo pulse sequence that was capable of collecting 32 echoes from seven 5-mm slices in less than 20 minutes. By adding gradient echoes on either side of the spin

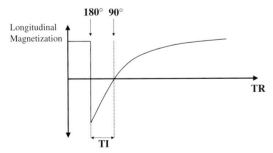

Fig. 3. Curve shows the recovery of longitudinal magnetization after an inversion pulse used to determine T1 relaxation time. In this particular case, TI was chosen at the magnetization null point.

echo, this three-dimensional sequence was shortened by a factor of between three and five.[42]

In any T2 measurement, it is important to collect images at as many TE times as possible to fully characterize the T2 decay curve. For brain with MS lesions, if one wishes to characterize all potential T2 components, images should be collected with TE times no longer than 10 milliseconds out to TE times more than 1 second.[43] For reliable results, the signal-to-noise ratio for the image with the shortest TE time should be at least 100:1.[44]

Analysis of T1 and T2 Relaxation Data

For single component T1 relaxation acquired with sufficiently long TR times, the signal follows:

$$S(TI) = S(TI = \infty)\left(1 - fe^{\frac{-TI}{T_1}}\right) \qquad (6)$$

where $S(TI = \infty)$ is the equilibrium signal achieved after a long pause (ie, no radiofrequency pulses) and f characterizes the efficiency of the inversion pulse. For a saturation recovery measurement, $f = 1$ and for an IR measurement with perfect 180° pulses, $f = 2$. If $S(TI = \infty)$ is known, one can fit a simpler exponential function:

$$S(TI) - S(TI = \infty) = S(TI = \infty)e^{\frac{-TI}{T_1}} \qquad (7)$$

For single component T2 relaxation, the T2 decay curve follows the same form:

$$S(TE) = S(TE = 0)e^{\frac{-TE}{T_2}} \qquad (8)$$

CNS tissue is inhomogeneous; consequently, analysis of relaxation time data from brain should be capable of distinguishing multiple components. This is especially true for T2 studies of brain and cord.[7] Analyses that estimate T2 times from images acquired at only two TE times are inappropriate. For monoexponential decay curves, two-point T2 estimations are susceptible to noise; for multiexponential decay curves, two-point T2 estimations depend critically on the chosen TE times.[45] For reliable T2 estimations in the presence of multi-component T2 relaxation, many more than two TE times are required.

For multi-component T2 relaxation, the T2 decay curve follows:

$$S(TE) = \sum S_i e^{\frac{-TE}{T_{2i}}} \qquad (9)$$

where S_i and T_{2i} relate to water component i. Multi-component T1 analyses can be handled with an equivalent modification of equation 8. Much literature (eg,[44,46–50]) discusses fitting multi-exponential relaxation decays. It is desirable, if not essential, to use an analysis that does not require a priori the number of contributing components. Many users

in the field[39,51–54] use the nonnegative least squares algorithm,[55] which inverts a relaxation decay curve to a relaxation time distribution. The relaxation time distribution is a plot of signal versus relaxation time. The nonnegative least squares algorithm uses χ^2 minimization to fit the relaxation decay curve to a large number of relaxation times. The nonnegative least squares algorithm produces a T2 distribution that consists of a few discrete spikes; however, most investigators prefer a smooth distribution. A continuous distribution can be achieved by minimizing χ^2 and a regularizer. A common regularizer is the sum of the squares of the solution amplitudes—the so-called "small model."[47] An example of a T2 distribution from brain tissue can be seen in **Fig. 5**.

Another approach to dealing with multi-component relaxation curves is to use nonlinear curve fitting techniques.[56–60] In many applications, researchers have simultaneously fit T1 and T2 relaxation times.[57,58,60] The nonlinear fitting approach requires more a priori information; however, if the a priori information is accurate, this approach may result in more robust solutions.

Measurement and Analysis of T2* Relaxation and Susceptibility-Weighted Imaging

For the measurement of T2*, the refocusing pulses of the spin echo sequence, which compensate for the T2′ decay, are omitted and the signal is sampled with several readout gradients (multi-echo gradient echo imaging). The challenge in measuring T2* is the separation of the tissue-specific decay from the decay caused by background field inhomogeneities. A simple and effective approach is to increase spatial resolution so that there is less

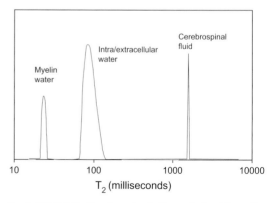

Fig. 5. T2 distribution from brain tissue derived from the nonnegative least squares algorithm for nonexponential decay curves. Three different water environments can be separated: myelin water, intra/extracellular water, and CSF.

variation in resonance frequency within a voxel.[27,28] Other methods are based on the assumption that the main contribution to the inhomogeneities arises from a constant background gradient along the through-plane direction, because slice thickness is usually larger than the in-plane dimensions of a voxel. Multiple scans with different compensation gradients can be acquired and combined[61] using postprocessing methods.[62] These methods can be aided by a map of the background field inhomogeneities.[63] Models for T2* signal behavior exist for vascular networks[19,64] and for single straight blood vessels.[19,23,24,65] In **Fig. 2**, the numerical simulation and the measured signal are shown for single blood vessels oriented parallel and perpendicular to the magnetic field.

Phase and magnitude are the two ingredients of SWI,[29,31,32] a gradient echo method that uses long TE together with high spatial resolution. The high spatial resolution reduces the sequence's sensitivity to background field inhomogeneities of the static magnetic field while maintaining or even increasing sensitivity to partial volume effects induced by small venous vessels or small structures with different magnetic susceptibility compared with their surroundings.[28,29] These susceptibility differences produce local field inhomogeneities that lead to a faster signal decay compared with magnetically homogeneous tissue. The inhomogeneities produced by a vein, for instance, reach far into the tissue surrounding the vein.[25] This effect allows visualization of veins much smaller than the voxel size. Veins with a diameter of approximately 200 µm are seen with a spatial resolution of 0.5 × 0.5 × 1 mm.[31] The magnetic field in a voxel also may experience an offset because of a constant and homogeneous but different tissue susceptibility, rather than field inhomogeneities. The sensitivity toward such offsets is maintained by incorporating phase.

MR signals and images can be represented by complex numbers that have magnitude and phase. The magnitude and the phase of voxels in T2*-weighted images bear complementary information. If the field variations have high spatial frequencies compared with the voxel size, intravoxel spin dephasing and accelerated T2′ decay occur. If the field variations have low spatial frequency, the field within a voxel can be regarded as constant, but the precession frequency still may be altered. This offset in resonance frequency becomes apparent in the phase of the signal:

$$\Delta\phi = -\gamma \bullet \Delta B \bullet TE \qquad (10)$$

where ΔB is the deviation from the static magnetic field B_0. The noise of a phase image is determined by the signal-to-noise ratio of the corresponding magnitude image and is independent of the actual phase angle.[66]

Phase information is acquired simultaneously with the magnitude of a T2*-weighted sequence. It is limited to values ranging from $-\pi$ to $+\pi$ and is periodic, resulting in aliasing of the true phase, often referred to as phase wrapping. The wrapped phase differs from the true phase by integer multiples of 2 π. Retrieving the true phase from the wrapped phase (phase unwrapping) can be difficult, especially in the presence of noise. Phase unwrapping is a common problem in the imaging sciences, and there are countless algorithms; several methods optimized for MRI data have been developed.[67–70]

The most common analysis used with SWI is to process three images: the magnitude, the phase, and a combination, in which the phase is converted into a mask and multiplied with the magnitude.[31] This mask enhances the contrast between small venous vessels and the surrounding parenchyma.

RESULTS FROM NORMAL BRAIN AND CORD
T1 Relaxation

T1 times in normal brain at 1.5 T are approximately 700 milliseconds (WM) to 1200 milliseconds (GM).[7] Most, but not all, of the literature suggests that on this timescale, brain water can be considered to act as a single component (ie, all water molecules have the same T1). The most important determinant of T1 in brain is water content.[71–76] A simple theory based on the assumption of fast exchange between bulk water and water closely associated with nonaqueous tissue gives an expression linking T1 and water content:[71]

$$\frac{1}{T_1} = A\left(\frac{1}{WC}\right) + B \qquad (11)$$

where A and B are constants and WC is the water content. This model, which is well supported by data in some studies,[73,77,78] explains why GM and MS lesions have longer T1 times than WM. Other studies demonstrate a linear relationship between 1/T1 and iron content, however. [79,80] In summary, for normal brain, T1 is dominated by water content, but this relationship also may be affected by iron content. More work is required to validate these relationships in MS.

Two recent studies challenged the conventional picture of T1 relaxation in brain by demonstrating multi-component T1 relaxation in normal brain. [81,82] These two studies highlighted the fact that the water and nonaqueous tissue are affected differently by MRI inversion pulses. Complete understanding of these interesting new results has not yet been achieved, and they present an exciting challenge to investigators in the field of CNS MRI.

T2 Relaxation

Fig. 3 shows T2 decay curves measured from pure water, NWM, normal GM, and an MS lesion. The decay curve from pure water is monoexponential and follows a straight line on the semi-logarithmic plot. Most decay curves from brain cannot be fit properly by a single exponential function, which suggests the existence of more than one water reservoir, each with its own T2 time. Decay curves from different WM and GM structures follow different trajectories.

A typical T2 distribution from brain tissue at 1.5 T is displayed in **Fig. 5**. Each peak corresponds to a different water environment; in the case of slow exchange, the relative areas under the peaks scale as the amount of water in each environment. The three T2 components in normal brain[7] are CSF with a long T2 over 2 seconds, intra- and extracellular water with an intermediate T2 of approximately 80 milliseconds, and water between the sheaths of the myelin bilayers with a short T2 of approximately 20 milliseconds. Unfortunately, with the currently available resolution of the T2 distribution, separation of the signals from intra- and extracellular water in normal brain is not possible. The intra- and extracellular water peak in the T2 distribution is commonly characterized by its geometric mean (ie, mean on a logarithmic scale).[7] The total area under the T2 distribution is proportional to the water content. If an external water standard is used and T1 weighting and temperature[83] is taken into account, the area under the T2 distribution can be used to measure absolute water content.[7] An alternative approach to measuring water content in brain is to extrapolate the T2* decay curve to TE = 0.[8] The assignment of the shortest T2 component to myelin water is supported by many studies of central and peripheral nervous system tissue dating back to 1969.[5,84–88] The myelin water fraction (MWF) is defined as the ratio of the area under the myelin water peak to the total area of the T2 distribution. Several in vitro studies using histopathologic identification of myelin demonstrated that the MWF is strongly correlated with myelin content.[51,89,90]

The MWF of GM is much smaller than that of WM. In brain, different WM structures have different MWF; for example, the MWF for the posterior internal capsules (approximately 16%) is more than twice as large as that from the minor forceps (approximately 5%).[7] Cord MWF values are larger than those in brain; typical MWFs in cord are 25%, although values do vary with anatomic level.[91–94] **Fig. 6** shows an example of a myelin water image from a healthy control.

A different approach to extracting the MWF is to derive a filter that produces either a myelin water image or a total water image when applied to a series of images acquired at different TE times. Using this novel approach, Jones and colleagues[95] and Vidarsson and colleagues[96] created myelin water images from a linear combination of as few as three echoes. This linear combination approach could lead to techniques for fast acquisition of myelin water images. With this technique, however, shifts in the T2 time of the myelin water caused by disease might be interpreted artifactually as decreases or increases in MWF.

The literature reports single component T1 relaxation and multi-component T2 relaxation in WM.[7] One can deduce that on the T2 timescale of approximately 100 milliseconds, myelin water remains in the myelin bilayers, but on the T1 timescale of approximately 1 second, myelin water exchanges with intra- and extracellular water. Several studies that explored this concept confirmed that myelin water exchange does occur on this intermediate time scale.[6,38,97] The rate of this exchange process should be temperature dependent; room temperature in vitro measurements of WM have identified different T1 times for the myelin water and intra- and extracellular water pools.[6,98] The current assumption is that MWF values are only slightly influenced by exchange processes, but more work is required before the effects of exchange on the T2 distribution are completely understood.[6]

In summary, T2 relaxation can provide MWF and total water content in normal brain and cord. These values differ for different regions in the brain and spinal cord. A representative MWF image is shown in **Fig. 6**.

T2* Relaxation and Susceptibility-Weighted Imaging

T2*
Peters and colleagues[99] determined T2* for different brain structures using a multi-echo planar imaging approach and the background field inhomogeneity correction suggested by Dahnke and Schaefter.[63] They found an approximately linear relationship between 1/T2* and field strength. T2* ranged from 26.8 ms ± 1.2 milliseconds (at 7.0 T) to 66.2 ± 1.9 milliseconds (at 1.5 T) in WM and from 33.2 ±1.3 milliseconds (at 7.0 T) to 84.0 ± 0.8 milliseconds (1.5 T) in cortical GM. In blood, T2 and T2* depend on the blood oxygenation. T2*

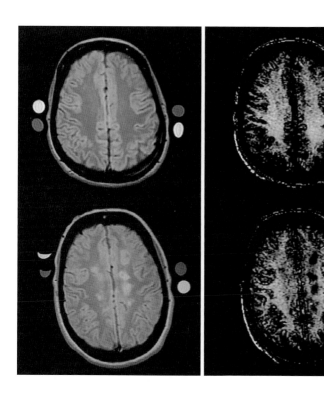

Fig. 6. Single slice proton density and MWF map (area under the curve of the short T2 component divided by the area for the total T2 distribution) from a healthy control (*top*) and from a patient who has MS (*bottom row*) acquired at 1.5 T using a 32 echo relaxation sequence.

values obtained at an oxygenation of 60% are 97 milliseconds at 1.5 T,[100] 21.2 milliseconds at 3 T,[101] and 7.4 ± 1.4 milliseconds at 7.0 T.[102] This blood oxygenation dependency of the MR signal is the basis of function MRI (fMRI).[30] Most BOLD fMRI studies use fast T2*-weighted imaging to investigate brain function.[103] Signal changes caused by neuronal activity measured with an echo planar imaging sequence (TE = 30 milliseconds, voxel size = 3 × 3 × 3 mm^3) are approximately 2.5% at 1.5 T and 4.5% at 3.0 T.[104]

Susceptibility-weighted imaging

Initially, SWI was developed with the aim of visualizing the cerebral venous architecture by exploiting the partial volume effect induced by veins, which leads to a faster signal decay than in homogeneous tissue (see **Fig. 2**).[29,105] At 1.5 T, SWI is usually performed with a TE of approximately 40 milliseconds, a flip angle of approximately 25°, and a spatial resolution of 0.5 × 0.5 × 2 mm.[106,107] The rather long TE can be shortened with a T1-reducing contrast agent,[108] which reduces data acquisition time and sensitivity to background field inhomogeneities. At 3.0 T, TEs of approximately 28 milliseconds were found to give good results.[109] Simulations and measurements at 7.0 T showed that an optimum T2* contrast between venous blood and brain tissue is obtained at TE = 15 milliseconds.[102]

That gradient echo images detect blood oxygenation changes associated with neural activation[103] has been demonstrated using flow compensated two- or three-dimensional methods.[110,111] Because the SWI technique is intrinsically BOLD sensitive, it can be used for functional imaging with high spatial resolution. Recently, SWI was used in combination with modulated blood oxygenation by inhalation of carbogen, a mixture of carbon dioxide and oxygen, and oxygen in imaging vascular function in healthy volunteers.[25] With SWI, the influence of large draining veins on the spatial properties of the BOLD response, for instance, has been demonstrated for the visual cortex.[112]

The potential value of the phase images as a measure of magnetic susceptibility was recognized early.[113,114] Magnetic susceptibility-weighted MR phase imaging provides a wealth of information because of small differences in the local resonance frequency.[115] After phase unwrapping in image space and high-pass filtering to remove the undesired effects from background field inhomogeneities, phase images display small anatomic structures with good contrast. Deep nuclei with increased iron content, small veins, and even WM tracts, which are not easily visible on corresponding magnitude images, become apparent in the phase (**Fig. 7**). Deistung and colleagues[116,117] demonstrated the magnetic fields

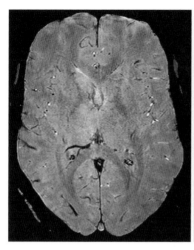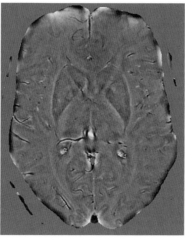

Fig. 7. Magnitude (*left*) and phase (*right*) of an SWI scan of a healthy volunteer (3 T, Philips Achieva, 8 channel head coil, TE = 21 milliseconds, TR = 28 milliseconds, $\alpha = 14°$).

produced by nearly spherical diamagnetic (calcifications) and paramagnetic lesions in the human brain. There is also increased contrast between cortical GM and WM, with phase images acquired at 7.0 T even displaying the cortical substructure.[118] Ogg and colleagues[119] demonstrated a correlation between phase shifts in gradient echo images and iron content of GM, but not in WM.[120] Similar findings were reported by Haacke and colleagues[121] in a study of six healthy volunteers, and recent work showed that there is a difference in the phase between hemispheres but not between genders.[122] Despite this progress, the source of contrast in susceptibility-weighted phase images is not well understood. Content of heme and non-heme iron alone, for instance, cannot explain the phase differences between GM and WM.[118] Recent work by Zhong and colleagues[123] suggested that the macromolecule content also may be responsible for the differences in phase between different tissues.

MULTIPLE SCLEROSIS
T1 Relaxation in Multiple Sclerosis

Lesions
The earliest relaxation study of MS[124] found that the T1 of acute lesions was higher than that of chronic lesions and the T1 of chronic lesions was higher than that of NWM. Over months, the T1 of acute lesions decreased to values matching the T1 of chronic lesions,[124] also confirmed by Larsson and colleagues[125] The T1 of lesions was found to be monexponential in all cases but showed a wide range of values likely because of differing lesion pathology.[125,126] Hypointense T1 lesions showed a longer T1 than MS lesions that are isointense on T1 images. The T1 of enhancing lesions

fell between the two values.[127] In most lesions, T1 was even more elevated than in normal-appearing WM (NAWM) likely because of the increase in water caused by edema and increased extracellular fluid spaces. The link between edema and T1 was justified by the strong correlation between T1 and water content in MS tissue.[128] However, in 8 of 151 lesions found in the posterior fossa in one study,[129] similar T1 and T2 values to NAWM made the lesions invisible on a fast FLAIR sequence.

Many studies have used T1-weighted images to detect lesions with abnormally long T1 compared with NAWM, known as hypointense T1 lesions or T1 black holes.[130] Whereas correlations between T2 lesion load and disability have been fairly weak,[131,132] stronger correlations have been found between hypointense T1 lesions load and disability,[130,133] between hypointense T1 lesions and recovery from relapses,[134] and between increases in hypointense T1 lesion load and progressive cerebral atrophy.[135] In larger follow-up studies, the correlation between disability and hypointense T1 lesions load was weaker although still significant.[136,137] In a 4-year serial study on nine patients who had MS, Bagnato and colleagues[138] found that 41% of contrast-enhancing lesions also showed T1 hypointensity and 22% of contrast-enhancing lesions continued to show T1 hypointensity after the contrast enhancement had stopped. Hypointense T1 lesions have lower levels of N-acetyl-aspartate (a marker of neuronal integrity) and increased concentration of choline (a membrane breakdown product),[139,140] increased T1, T2 and water content,[127] and increased apparent diffusion coefficient and decreased diffusion anisotropy.[141–144] Early work on biopsy samples of MS tissue showed a correlation between the degree of hypointensity and the extent of axonal damage, extracellular edema, demyelination, and remyelination.[145] In a postmortem study of five brains affected by MS, the degree of hypointensity was not correlated with degree of demyelination or the number of reactive astrocytes but was well correlated with axonal density.[146] This close association with T1 hypointensity and axonal content was confirmed by van Waesberghe and colleagues[147] in postmortem MS tissue. In a longitudinal study that used brain biopsy for pathologic correlation, lesions were found to become more T1 hypointense in initially demyelinating lesions, but as remyelination occurred the T1 hypointensity decreased.[148] The extent of the observed increase in hypointensity was found to correlate highly with axonal loss.[148]

Normal-appearing white matter

Most studies on MS have found an increase in T1 times within NAWM compared with NWM.[129,149–158] These differences are more apparent supratentorially than infratentorially.[129] Although it was first thought that changes in T1 were from discrete areas of a few pixels,[154] later studies showed a global shift of the whole brain average T1 in MS indicating diffuse abnormalities (**Fig. 8**).[159,160] One study that compared secondary progressive MS (SPMS) and relapsing remitting MS (RRMS) only found significant differences in T1 between NWM and NAWM in SPMS.[155] In another study of early RRMS, however, the T1 of NAWM and GM were significantly higher than NWM.[156] Previous work found that T1 times for NAWM in the immediate vicinity of a lesion were higher than T1 times from NAWM remote from a lesion.[155]

T1 histograms

Because changes in MS occur over the entire brain, studying only lesions or specific regions may miss important results. Recently, histograms have been used to study entire slices or the whole brain.[158,161] In patients who had MS, the histogram peak position was found to occur at longer T1 than for controls.[156–159,162–164] T1 peak position was significantly higher in patients who had SPMS than RRMS or primary progressive MS (PPMS), and this increase was limited to WM, cortical GM, and the thalamus.[159] Vrenken and colleagues[165] found that T1 histogram peak heights for NAWM in SPMS and RRMS were reduced relative to those for NWM (**Fig. 8**). For individual voxels, in RRMS the T1 of 16% of NAWM voxels was increased compared with NWM; this value rose to 49% in SPMS.[159,160] In PPMS, this value was much smaller—only 1.5%. In longitudinal studies

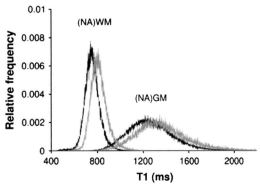

Fig. 8. Individual normalized unsmoothed histograms of cerebral normal-appearing (NA) WM (*left peaks*) and cerebral cortical normal-appearing GM (*right peaks*) of a patient who has MS (*gray lines*) and a healthy control subject (*black lines*) for comparison. Histogram peaks have symmetric near-normal shape, with clear separation of normal- appearing WM from normal appearing GM. (*From* Vrenken H, Geurts JJ, Knol DL, et al. Whole-brain T1 mapping in multiple sclerosis: global changes of normal-appearing gray and white matter. Radiology 2006;240:815; with permission.)

of RRMS and SPMS[157] and PPMS,[164] a significant increase in mean T1 and peak position and decrease in peak height were found in NAWM over time. In early RRMS, however, the only detectable change in the T1 histogram over 3 years was a small change in peak height.[156]

Mean T1 times and T1 histogram peak heights were a predictor of disability at 2 years,[164] and the mean T1 of NAWM correlated with disability.[157] Parry and colleagues[163] also found an inverse correlation between T1 histogram peak height from NAWM and disease duration. For specific WM tracts separated using DTI tractography, only the T1 from the corticospinal tract showed correlation with disability,[166] whereas the corpus callosum and total WM did not. Median WM T1 was found to correlate with supratentorial volume, lateral ventricle volume, and T2 lesion volume but not clinical parameters.[167] T1 histogram parameters were found to be strongly correlated with hypointense T1 lesion volume and atrophy,[162] which were related to progression of disease.

In a combined T1 and proton MR spectroscopy (^{1}H-MRS) study of parietal MS lesions in 11 patients who had SPMS, Brex and colleagues[168] found good correlations between T1 times and concentrations of total N-acetyl-aspartate and myo-inositol. They concluded that long T1 times correspond to low total N-acetyl-aspartate that results from severe axonal loss and to high myo-inositol, which is related to gliosis.

Spinal Cord

An increase in T1 in cervical cord has been measured in patients who have MS compared with controls.[169] T1 was significantly greater in cervical cord from patients who had SPMS compared with patients who had RRMS.[169] The median cervical cord T1 was correlated with median cerebral WM T1, upper cervical cord area, and the Expanded Disability Status Scale score.[169] In a postmortem study of spinal cord, T1 time was correlated with myelin content and axonal density.[170]

T_2 Relaxation in Multiple Sclerosis

Lesions

The earliest use of T2 relaxation in the study of MS was also by Ormerod and colleagues.[124] Their serial study of MS demonstrated that although lesions showed increases in T2 compared with control WM, acute lesions had longer T2 than chronic lesions. Over time, the T2 of acute lesions decreased to the chronic lesion values, similar to T1 behavior. In another serial study, Larsson and colleagues[125] followed acute lesions and found T2 to be elevated but monoexponential. On follow-up, the T2 became biexponential in some lesions, mainly in the lesion center. After more time, these lesions showed decreases in T2 and reverted to monoexponential relaxation. Goodkin and colleagues[171] and Vavasour and colleagues,[172] using a 32-echo T2 measurement, also found that new lesions showed increases in T2 that returned toward prelesion values at later months, although the T2 never returned to NAWM values.

In two studies, 7 of 33[126] and 28 of 53[173] chronic MS lesions were found to have biexponential T2 relaxation. In a larger study,[56] 87% of lesions were found to have biexponential T2 decay, with the shorter component between 50 and 120 milliseconds and the longer T2 component between 150 and 560 milliseconds. Over time, changes in T2 relaxation were found to be associated with changes in the long T2 component (> 300 milliseconds). These areas were identified as regions with CSF, blood-brain barrier breakdown, and edema.[56] In 13 patients who had MS, biexponential T2 was most common in T1 black holes and enhancing lesions.[174] Fewer biexponential T2 fits were found for diffusely abnormal WM, NAWM, or mildly hypointense T1 lesions, and no biexponential fits were needed for nonenhancing isointense T1 lesions or NWM.

Recently, a longer T2 component (200 milliseconds < T2 < 800 milliseconds) was detected using a 48-echo sequence, with the first 32 echoes at 10-millisecond spacing and the last 16 echoes at 50-millisecond spacing. In 20 patients who had MS, this long T2 component was detected in 23 of 97 lesions from 50% of the patients.[43] Lesions possessing a long T2 component also had higher water contents, longer mean T2 and T1, lower MWF, and lower MT ratio (MTR). Patients who had MS with lesions with the long T2 component also had significantly longer disease duration than patients who did not.

Two studies used 16 echoes and either monoexponential or biexponential fitting to separate different MS phenotypes. Filippi and colleagues[175] found that 75% of lesions from patients who had SPMS were biexponential compared with only 12.5% of lesions being biexponential in patients who had benign MS. In a larger study by Kidd and colleagues[176] of 40 patients who had MS, the most frequent biexponential lesions were found in PPMS lesions at 50%, whereas other MS subtypes were less frequent (benign: 23%; RR: 30%; SP: 29%).

Using a 32-echo T2 sequence,[177] 189 lesions were examined in 33 patients who had MS. Compared with contralateral NAWM, on average these lesions had 52% lower MWF and 5.8% higher water content. **Fig. 6** shows an example of a myelin map from a patient who has MS. Using a 12-echo, eight-slice T2 sequence in a study of 89 patients who had MS,[178] mean MWF of nonenhancing lesions was decreased to 8.4% and in enhancing lesions reduced to 8.0% compared with NAWM MWF values of 11.3%.[178] In a study of seven patients who had MS, chronic isointense and hypointense T1 lesions had similar MWF, although both were significantly lower than NAWM.[127] Lesions less than 1 year old had higher MWF than lesions more than 1 year old.[127] In a study of 10 patients who had MS, Stevenson and colleagues[129] found that T1 and T2 relaxation times of infratentorial lesions were close to the relaxation times of local NAWM, which resulted in reduced contrast between posterior fossa lesions and the background NAWM.

Normal-appearing white matter

In an early study of patients who had chronic MS, Larsson and colleagues[126] found that T2 was elevated in NAWM but fit a monoexponential curve, whereas T2 was biexponential in almost all cortical GM regions, which was attributed to partial volume effects with CSF. In another study,[56] some NAWM regions were found to have biexponential T2 decay. As with T1, differences in T2 in NAWM were first thought to arise from small lesions of one or two pixels in size.[154] In later studies, T2 times in NAWM were found to be shifted globally relatively to NWM histograms, and not just in small regions.[179,180] The NAWM from the genu and splenium of the corpus callosum showed the largest increase in mean T2 compared with NWM, although all NAWM regions showed a much larger variation in T2 than NWM.[179,180] Using T2 histograms of WM, Grenier and colleagues[180] were able to differentiate patients who had MS from controls and RRMS from SPMS and PPMS.

Using a single-slice 32-echo T2 sequence, a study at 1.5 T on 33 patients who had MS found that the mean water content of NAWM was 2.2% higher than in NWM and the mean MWF was 16% lower.[177] The decrease in MWF was modeled as diffuse myelin loss throughout the NAWM. In an eight-slice, 12-echo study at 3.0 T, a cohort of 89 patients and 28 controls were found to have an average MWF for NAWM and NWM of 10.6% and 11.3%, respectively.[178] If patients were divided into groups with a disease duration of less than or more than 5 years, MWF was found to be 10.8% and 10.3%, respectively. Note that these two MWF studies examined different brain regions.

Goodkin and colleagues[171] found that regions of NAWM that developed lesions had elevated T2 compared with regions of NAWM that did not develop into lesions. Prelesional changes in measurements from NAWM have been found in magnetization transfer imaging,[171,181–183] 1H-MRS,[184] and DTI.[185]

Spinal cord

The mean T2 relaxation times from demyelinating lesions in the cervical spinal cord were found to be similar to values from normal controls, but the MWF was significantly lower.[91] Lower MWFs were also found in a study of 24 patients who had PPMS compared with matched controls.[93] After 2 years, a significant decrease in MWF was observed in patients who had MS but not in controls.

Ex vivo studies

In a postmortem study of spinal cord, Mottershead and colleagues[170] found that mean T2 correlated only moderately with myelin content and axonal count but correlated more strongly with other MR measures. Other measures derived from the T2 distribution, such as MWF, have been found to be specific to pathology, however. Histopathologic validation of the MWF as a marker for myelin in human WM comes from qualitative and quantitative comparison of MWF with the anatomic distribution of myelin as shown with luxol fast blue stain.[89,90,186] On 37 fixed brain slices imaged and subsequently stained for luxol fast blue, the average R^2 between MWF and luxol fast blue optical density was 0.67 at 1.5 T[89] and 0.78 at 7.0 T,[90] which showed evidence that MWF is a validated

marker for myelin in WM. **Fig. 9** shows an example of the qualitative and quantitative correspondence between luxol fast blue and MWF.

Using an NMR spectrometer and 124-echo T2 experiments with echo delays varying from 2 μs to 144 milliseconds, Ramani and colleagues[187] investigated fixed WM slices of normal and MS brain. They distinguished three components in the decay curves: a rapidly decaying signal, presumably arising from protons on nonaqueous molecules, an intermediate component with T2 of a few milliseconds, and a larger component with T2 of approximately 15 milliseconds. The latter component had a T2 time similar to that of myelin water in vivo. Surprisingly, this study did not reveal a longer T2 component with T2 of 40 to 60 milliseconds corresponding to intra- and extracellular water; such a component was found in other formalin fixed brain experiments. The relative amount of the initial rapidly decaying signal was decreased substantially in samples from MS brain, consistent with demyelination.[187]

T2* and Susceptibility-Weighted Imaging in Multiple Sclerosis

By minimizing the T2' decay, Du and colleagues[59] were able to use gradient echo imaging to assess myelin content in vitro via the characteristic T2 decay of myelin water. With a fast gradient echo method, the first echo was sampled at 2 milliseconds and the echo spacing was only 1 millisecond, which allowed sampling of the myelin water signal with a high temporal rate. The MWF obtained with this technique was in good agreement with previous results.[7,95,177]

Tan and colleagues[188] performed BOLD MR venography in 17 subjects who had MS with SWI and found that all but 1 of the 95 MS lesions were traversed by a vein. Shape and orientation of the lesions corresponded well with the veins. Similar results were obtained recently at 7 T in a study of 89 lesions in 10 patients, in whom 82% of the lesions were associated with veins.[189] Association with veins was more likely in periventricular (96%) than in peripheral lesions (65%). Haacke and colleagues[190] found that many lesions seen in SWI were not seen with T2-weighted images, whereas Eissa and colleagues[191] came to the opposite conclusion. An explanation for this discrepancy may be that in the study by Eissa and colleagues, the spatial resolution was much higher for T2-weighted imaging than for SWI. An investigation of phase images acquired with a standard gradient echo sequence in ten patients who had MS found heterogeneous patterns of phase hypointensities.[192] Shah and colleagues[193] found in ten

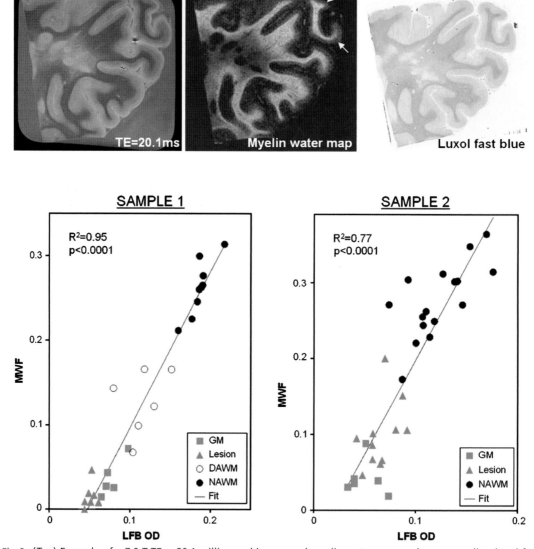

Fig. 9. (*Top*) Example of a 7.0-T TE = 20.1 millisecond image and myelin water map and corresponding luxol fast blue histology image of the parieto-occipital region of a patient who has MS. A good qualitative correspondence is observed between the myelin water map and histology stain for myelin. The normal prominent myelination of the deeper cortical layers (*arrows*) is also visible on the myelin water image. (*Bottom*) Examples of the quantitative correlation between myelin water fraction (MWF) and luxol fast blue optical density (LFB OD) for gray matter (GM), lesion, dirty-appearing white matter (DAWM), and normal-appearing white matter (NAWM) for two MS samples. (*From* Laule C, Kozlowski P, Leung E, Myelin water imaging of multiple sclerosis at 7 T: correlations with histopathology. Neuroimage 2008;40:1577–78; with permission.)

patients investigated at 7.0 T that out of 255 lesions seen in the magnitude image, only 140 were visible as hypointensities in the phase image and that most lesions were associated with small veins. **Fig. 10** shows an example of magnitude, phase, and SWI images from a patient who had MS.[191]

Although fMRI is based on changes in T2 and T2* caused by neural activity, an in-depth discussion of fMRI in MS is beyond the scope of this article, and we refer readers to the existing literature[194–196] and to the article by Filippi and Rocca elsewhere in this issue.

Exogeneous Contrast Agents in Multiple Sclerosis

The use of Gd-based contrast agents for monitoring blood-brain barrier breakdown through

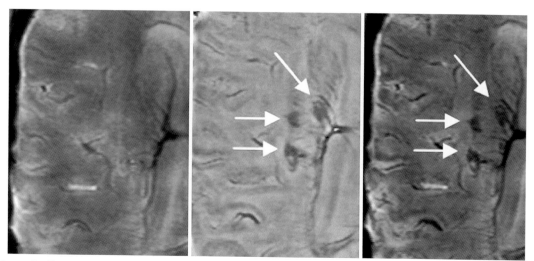

Fig. 10. (*Left*) Magnitude, (*center*) phase, (*right*) SWI of a 66-year-old patient with MS lesions visible (*arrows*) in the phase (*center*) but not in the magnitude (*left*). (*From* Eissa A, Lebel R, Korzan J, et al. MRI of multiple sclerosis with high contrast susceptibility-weighting and extreme resolution T2-weighting. Presented at ISMRM. Toronto, Canada, 2008; with permission.)

manipulating T1, T2, and T2* is well established in clinical MR of patients who have MS. Recently, this field has blossomed with the advent of targeted agents and agents based on super paramagnetic iron oxide particles.[197] In an animal model, a targeted Gd-based agent was demonstrated to attach to selectin, which is associated with endothelial activation in brain inflammation.[198] Using another Gd-targeted agent, Wessig and colleagues[199] specifically labeled nerve fibers undergoing demyelination.

Super paramagnetic iron oxide particles have yielded exciting new information about the inflammatory process in vivo in patients who have MS.[200–202] Vellinga and colleagues[200] and Dousset and colleagues[201] demonstrated that ultra-small super paramagnetic iron oxide particles behave differently than Gd agents and provide more insight in the pluriformity of inflammation in MS. Ultrasmall super paramagnetic iron oxide contrast was found to indicate macrophage activity and predict lesion severity in relapsing EAE.[203] These iron oxide agents are sensitive; single-cell imaging has been confirmed in animal studies.[202,204–206]

COMPARISON WITH OTHER MRI TECHNIQUES
T2 Relaxation and Diffusion

To better interpret the results of relaxation experiments in normal human brain and in brain affected by MS, it is useful to compare findings with metrics from other MRI techniques. DTI has become a popular tool for studying MS because various metrics obtained from DTI are thought to reflect

the integrity of myelin or axons. Water in WM diffuses preferentially along the primary direction of axons rather than perpendicular to them; the diffusion tensor is much more anisotropic in WM than in GM, where there are fewer impediments to diffusion on the timescale of the diffusion experiment.[207,208] A commonly cited measure of diffusion anisotropy is fractional anisotropy (FA), defined as the ratio of the standard deviation of the diffusion tensor to its mean principal value; FA has a value between 0 (when diffusion is perfectly isotropic) and 1 (for diffusion restricted entirely to one direction). In the presence of myelin, water is expected to be more strongly restricted to the direction of the neurons; hence, FA should decrease with myelin damage. FA can be an ambiguous measure because decreases could be caused by a reduction of lateral restriction or simply an increase in diffusion parallel to fiber tracts; the diffusion tensor eigenvalues have been proposed as more specific measures of pathology.[209–211] The largest eigenvalue, $\lambda_{\parallel}$, is the diffusivity parallel to the dominant diffusion direction and is thought to reflect axonal integrity, whereas the average of the two smaller eigenvalues, $\lambda_{\perp}$, is the diffusivity perpendicular to the prevailing direction of diffusion, which has been linked to myelin pathology.[212–220]

Normal Brain

FA has been shown to be correlated with MWF in healthy CNS tissue.[221,222] Different brain structures deviate from the relationship, however. For example, although the genu of the corpus callosum and major forceps have similar MWF values, they differ significantly in terms of FA because of the difference in degree of fiber organization. **Fig. 11** shows a comparison between MWF and FA in a region of crossing fibers from Mädler and colleagues.[221] It has been shown that whereas FA values are affected by myelin, they are primarily determined by intact axonal membranes.[223]

Similar correlations have been observed between $\lambda_\perp$ and MWF,[221,222] with smaller values of $\lambda_\perp$ observed for large MWFs; however, $\lambda_\perp$ is also affected by the degree of organization of fibers and is increased in areas of crossing fibers. Because myelin and axons are expected to correlate in healthy tissue, a relationship between MWF and $\lambda_\parallel$ also could be anticipated. Although a correlation was found between $\lambda_\parallel$ and MWF by Mädler and colleagues ($R^2 = 0.55$), no correlation was found by Bells and colleagues[222] ($R^2 = 0.05$). $\lambda_\parallel$ does not vary greatly in healthy CNS tissue; thus the smaller selection of regions of interest in the Bells study may have rendered any relationship insignificant.

Brain Affected by Multiple Sclerosis

The relationship between MWF and DTI metrics that was observed in normal CNS tissue breaks down in MS pathology.[224] In NAWM, no correlation was observed between MWF and FA, $\lambda_\perp$, or $\lambda_\parallel$. Although a large range of MWF values was observed in NAWM, DTI metrics did not vary much in the regions measured. In lesions in which a larger range of values was observed for DTI measures, a weak correlation was observed between MWF and $\lambda_\perp$. If only lesions with a long T2 component (with T2 between 200 and 800 milliseconds) were considered, however, much stronger correlations were observed between MWF and $\lambda_\perp$ and $\lambda_\parallel$. A weak correlation was also found with FA. Lesions with a long T2 component showed the greatest variation in DTI metric values. $\lambda_\perp$ was found to increase for low MWFs, which is consistent with findings in animal models, indicating that changes in $\lambda_\perp$ are linked to myelin integrity.[212,213,215–217,219] $\lambda_\parallel$ was found to increase for low MWF values, contrary to animal studies in which $\lambda_\parallel$ decreased with axonal damage,[215,217–219] but it was consistent with studies in which $\lambda_\parallel$ was found to increase with myelin damage,[213,225,226] attributed to decreased extra-axonal diffusion restrictions caused by either an absence of compact myelin or an increase in the partial volume of cell bodies within the regions of interest.

Although MWF and diffusion anisotropy measures offer information related to the amount and state of myelin and axons within a region of the brain, this information is not redundant but complementary. MWF seems to be more sensitive to changes in MS pathology.

RELAXATION AND MAGNETIZATION TRANSFER

MT measures exchange of magnetization between mobile protons on water and nonaqueous protons on macromolecules (eg, myelin). By applying an off-resonance pulse, the magnetization from

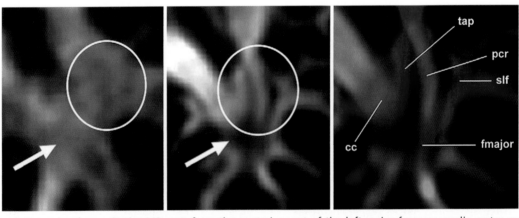

Fig. 11. Example of quantitative MR map from the posterior part of the left major forceps: myelin-water map (*left*), FA map (*middle*), and directional color coded FA map (*right*). Note the reduction of FA in the center of the major forceps (*arrow*). The two lines of reduced FA are caused by partial volume effects and separated fiber pathways between the superior and inferior longitudinal fasciculus (*slf*), and the tapetum (*tap*) merging with the major forceps (*fmajor*). They are not apparent in the myelin-water maps. (For interpretation of the references to color in this figure legend, the reader is referred to the Web version of this article.) (*From* Mädler B, Drabycz SA, Kolind SH, et al. Is diffusion anisotropy an accurate monitor of myelination? Correlation of multicomponent T2 relaxation and diffusion tensor anisotropy in human brain? Magnetic Resonance Imaging. 2008;26:874–88; with permission.)

non–MR-visible protons on macromolecules can be saturated; subsequent exchange with MRI visible protons on water can be seen as a decrease in signal. Often this exchange is characterized by an MT ratio, MTR = $(M_o-M_s)/M_o$, where M_s and M_o are the MR signal with and without the applied MT pulse. A decrease in MTR, which is often observed in MS tissue, can occur from either an increase in water content (eg, edema) or a decrease in the macromolecular pool (eg, demyelination or axonal loss).

T1 and Magnetization Transfer

A few studies have compared MTR with T1 relaxation in patients who have MS. 1/T1 and MTR were found to correlate strongly in lesions.[227] The strong correlation in lesions was also found by Griffin and colleagues,[228] but only a weak correlation and no correlation were found in NAWM and NWM, respectively. In postmortem brain, MTR was correlated with 1/T1.[229] Using quantitative MT, the MTR was found to best correlate with T_{1free}—the native T1 relaxation time—in severely hypointense T1 lesions but was also correlated in "dirty" or "diffusively abnormal" WM.[230]

T2 and Magnetization Transfer

T2 relaxation times were correlated with MTR in MS lesions, with the best correlation in hypointense T1 lesions[174] No significant correlation was found in NAWM or NWM; however, relaxation curves were fit to a monoexponential function in most cases. MTR often has been claimed to be a marker of myelin because myelin contributes to the nonaqueous proton pool. Myelin only makes up 50% of the nonaqueous component of WM,[3] however, and MTR depends highly on changes in water content. If MTR did measure myelin, then a correlation between MTR and MWF would be found. In MS lesions, only weak or no correlations have been observed between MWF and MTR in NWM, NAWM, and lesions.[52,231–233] Comparing quantitative MT and 32-echo T2 relaxation, no correlation between the semi-solid proton fraction (f_b) and the MWF was observed in NAWM, but a weak correlation was measured in lesions.[54]

Combined Magnetization Transfer and T2

If an off-resonance MT pulse is applied before the T2 relaxation sequence, the MT effect can be measured separately on the different water compartments. When the relaxation sequence was applied immediately after the MT pulse, the myelin water peak gave rise to an MTR twice that of the intra- and extracellular water peak.[38] As the delay time between the MT and T2 sequence was increased, the MTR of both peaks became the same, which indicated diffusion between the water compartments. This measurement provided an estimate of the lifetime of a water molecule within myelin to be on the order of several hundred milliseconds.[38] Another experiment of this type showed that exchange between the water compartments had more influence on MTR than on T2 relaxation times and amplitudes.[97] Exchange time between CSF and intra- and extracellular water pools has been measured using a combined sequence and found to be greater in NAWM than in lesions indicating more severe damage and increased extracellular spaces within lesions.[234]

SUMMARY

Dating back to the earliest days of clinical MRI, many research studies have been dedicated to the investigation of MR relaxation times in brain and cord affected by MS. A few common issues arise from this large body of knowledge. Water content plays a large role in determining T1 and T2 times. Water content also plays a large role in the pathologic process of MS. Generally speaking, the capability of T1 and T2 times to elucidate MS pathologies rests on the link between water content and pathology. To date, an insufficient number of studies have measured water content directly, partly because in vivo water content measurement is difficult.[4,5,7,8] Another confound might be the presence of iron, which also can influence T1 and T2 times; however, at least one study documented a correlation between iron and brain water content.[79,80]

For the many reasons discussed earlier in this article, it is challenging to measure relaxation times accurately, especially T2. Even if one could measure relaxation times quickly and accurately, at the current stage of our understanding of this field, it is not possible to attribute changes in relaxation times (especially T2) to specific pathologic changes. It seems that we should treat absolute relaxation times as qualitative numbers. In some cases, changes of relaxation times (eg, after addition of a contrast agent)[235] can be treated quantitatively.

Normal brain and cord contain multiple water compartments that are only slowly exchanging water on the T2 time scale. A T2 measurement includes not only T2 times but also relative compartment sizes. In this situation, although T2 times do not directly indicate pathology, the relative compartment sizes may relate to MS pathology (eg, the case of myelin water). There is a caveat in all multiple component systems, however: the rate of exchange between compartments should be slow on the MR measurement time scale so that measured component amplitudes are not affected by exchange.

SWI has been introduced to the MS field recently. Because it is somewhat specific for heme and non-heme iron, it promises to help define the role of veins and iron products in MS.

REFERENCES

1. Callaghan PT. Principles of nuclear magnetic resonance scopy. Oxford: Oxford University Press; 1991.
2. Bloembergen N, Purcell EM, Pound RV. Relaxation effects in nuclear magnetic resonance absorption. Physical Review 1948;73(7):679–712.
3. Norton W, Cammer W. Isolation and characterization of myelin. In: Morell P, editor. Myelin. 2nd edition. New York: Plenum Press; 1984. p. 147–95.
4. Fischer HW, Van Haverbeke Y, Schmitz-Feuerhake I, et al. The uncommon longitudinal relaxation dispersion of human brain white matter. Magn Reson Med 1989;9(3):441–6.
5. Stewart WA, MacKay AL, Whittall KP, et al. Spin-spin relaxation in experimental allergic encephalomyelitis: analysis of CPMG data using a non-linear least squares method and linear inverse theory. Magn Reson Med 1993;29(6):767–75.
6. Bjarnason T, Vavasour I, Chia C, et al. Characterization of the NMR behaviour of white matter in bovine brain. Magn Reson Med 2005;54:1072–81.
7. Whittall KP, MacKay AL, Graeb DA, et al. In vivo measurement of T2 distributions and water contents in normal human brain. Magn Reson Med 1997;37(1):34–43.
8. Neeb H, Zilles K, Shah NJ. A new method for fast quantitative mapping of absolute water content in vivo. Neuroimage 2006;31(3):1156–68.
9. Ye FQ, Martin WR, Allen PS. Estimation of brain iron in vivo by means of the interecho time dependence of image contrast. Magn Reson Med 1996;36(1):153–8.
10. Schenker C, Meier D, Wichmann W, et al. Age distribution and iron dependency of the T2 relaxation time in the globus pallidus and putamen. Neuroradiology 1993;35(2):119–24.
11. Einstein A. Motion of suspended particles in stationary liquids required from the molecular kinetic theory of heat. Annales der Physik 1905;17:549–60.
12. Hawkins CP, Munro PM, MacKenzie F, et al. Duration and selectivity of blood-brain barrier breakdown in chronic relapsing experimental allergic encephalomyelitis studied by gadolinium-DTPA and protein markers. Brain 1990;113(Pt 2):365–78.
13. Felix R, Laniado M, Claussen C, et al. Characterization of gadolinium-DTPA: basic properties and first clinical results. Presented at the 7th Carvat. Rome, Italy, February 6–10, 1984.
14. Ge Y, Law M, Johnson G, et al. Dynamic susceptibility contrast perfusion MR imaging of multiple sclerosis lesions: characterizing hemodynamic impairment and inflammatory activity. AJNR Am J Neuroradiol 2005;26(6):1539–47.
15. Schenck JF. The role of magnetic susceptibility in magnetic resonance imaging: MRI magnetic compatibility of the first and second kinds. Med Phys 1996;23(6):815–50.
16. Schenck JF. Safety of strong, static magnetic fields. J Magn Reson Imaging 2000;12(1):2–19.
17. Schenck JF, Zimmerman EA. High-field magnetic resonance imaging of brain iron: birth of a biomarker? NMR Biomed 2004;17(7):433–45.
18. Haacke EM, Cheng NYC, House MJ, et al. Imaging iron stores in the brain using magnetic resonance imaging. Magn Reson Imaging 2005;23(1):1–25.
19. Yablonskiy DA, Haacke EM. Theory of NMR signal behavior in magnetically inhomogeneous tissues: the static dephasing regime. Magn Reson Med 1994;32(6):749–63.
20. Pintaske J, Muller-Bierl B, Schick F. Geometry and extension of signal voids in MR images induced by aggregations of magnetically labelled cells. Phys Med Biol 2006;51(18):4707–18.
21. Brown RJS. Distribution of fields from randomly placed dipoles: free-precession signal decay as result of magnetic grains. Physical Review 1961; 121(5):1379–82.
22. Johnson MA, Li DK, Bryant DJ, et al. Magnetic resonance imaging: serial observations in multiple sclerosis. AJNR Am J Neuroradiol 1984;5(5):495–9.
23. Sedlacik J, Rauscher A, Reichenbach JR. Obtaining blood oxygenation levels from MR signal behavior in the presence of single venous vessels. Magn Reson Med 2007;58(5):1035–44.
24. Ziener CH, Bauer WR, Jakob PM. Frequency distribution and signal formation around a vessel. MAGMA 2005;18(4):225–30.
25. Rauscher A, Sedlacik J, Barth M, et al. Noninvasive assessment of vascular architecture and function during modulated blood oxygenation using susceptibility weighted magnetic resonance imaging. Magn Reson Med 2005;54(1):87–95.
26. Chu SC, Xu Y, Balschi JA, et al. Bulk magnetic susceptibility shifts in NMR studies of compartmentalized samples: use of paramagnetic reagents. Magn Reson Med 1990;13(2):239–62.
27. Young IR, Cox IJ, Bryant DJ, et al. The benefits of increasing spatial resolution as a means of reducing artifacts due to field inhomogeneities. Magn Reson Imaging 1988;6(5):585–90.

28. Haacke EM, Tkach JA, Parrish TB. Reduction of T2* dephasing in gradient field-echo imaging. Radiology 1989;170(2):457–62.

29. Reichenbach JR, Venkatesan R, Yablonskiy DA, et al. Theory and application of static field inhomogeneity effects in gradient-echo imaging. J Magn Reson Imaging 1997;7(2):266–79.

30. Ogawa S, Lee TM, Nayak AS, et al. Oxygenation-sensitive contrast in magnetic resonance image of rodent brain at high magnetic fields. Magn Reson Med 1990;14(1):68–78.

31. Reichenbach JR, Haacke EM. High-resolution BOLD venographic imaging: a window into brain function. NMR Biomed 2001;14(7–8):453–67.

32. Haacke EM, Xu Y, Cheng Y-CN, et al. Susceptibility weighted imaging (SWI). Magn Reson Med 2004;52(3):612–8.

33. Look DC, Locker DR. Time saving in measurement of NMR and EPR relaxation times. Rev Sci Instrum 1970;41:250–1.

34. Carr HY, Purcell EM. Effects of diffusion on free precession in nuclear magnetic resonance experiments. Physical Review 1954;94:630–9.

35. Meiboom G, Gill D. Modified spin echo method for measuring relaxation times. Rev Sci Instrum 1958;29:688–91.

36. Stefanovic B, Pike GB. Human whole-blood relaxometry at 1.5 T: assessment of diffusion and exchange models. Magn Reson Med 2004;52(4):716–23.

37. Poon CS, Henkelman RM. Practical T2 quantitation for clinical applications. J Magn Reson Imaging 1992;2(5):541–53.

38. Vavasour IM, Whittall KP, Li DK, et al. Different magnetization transfer effects exhibited by the short and long T(2) components in human brain. Magn Reson Med 2000;44(6):860–6.

39. Oh J, Han ET, Pelletier D, et al. Measurement of in vivo multi-component T2 relaxation times for brain tissue using multi-slice T2 prep at 1.5 and 3 T. Magn Reson Imaging. 2006;24(1):33–43.

40. Wright GA, Brittain JH, Stainsby JA. Preserving T1 or T2 contrast in magnetization preparation sequences. Presented at the 4th Annual Meeting of the International Society for Magnetic Resonance in Medicine. New York, 1996.

41. Mädler B, MacKay AL. In-vivo 3D multi-component T2-relaxation measurements for quantitative myelin imaging at 3T. Presented at the 14th Annual Meeting of the International Society of Magnetic Resonance in Medicine. Seattle, WA, 2006.

42. Mädler B, MacKay AL. Towards whole brain myelin imaging. Presented at the 15th Annual Meeting of the International Society for Magnetic Resonance in Medicine. Berlin, Germany, 2007.

43. Laule C, Vavasour IM, Kolind SH, et al. Long T2 water in multiple sclerosis: what else can we learn from multi-echo T2 relaxation? J Neurol 2007;254(11):1579–87.

44. Graham SJ, Stanchev PL, Bronskill MJ. Criteria for analysis of multicomponent tissue T2 relaxation data. Magn Reson Med 1996;35(3):370–8.

45. Whittall KP, MacKay AL, Li DK. Are mono-exponential fits to a few echoes sufficient to determine T2 relaxation for in vivo human brain? Magn Reson Med 1999;41(6):1255–7.

46. Provencher SW. A constrained regularization method for inverting data represented by linear algebraic or integral equations. Comput Phys Commun 1982;27:213–27.

47. Whittall KP, MacKay AL. Quantitative interpretation of NMR relaxation data. J Magn Reson 1989;84:134–52.

48. Fenrich FR, Beaulieu C, Allen PS. Relaxation times and structures. NMR Biomed 2001;14(2):133–9.

49. Kroeker RM, Henkelman RM. Analysis of biological NMR relaxation data with continuous distributions of relaxation times. J Magn Reson 1986;69:218–35.

50. Henkelman RM. Measurement of signal intensities in the presence of noise in MR images. Med Phys 1985;12(2):232–3.

51. Webb S, Munro CA, Midha R, et al. Is multicomponent T2 a good measure of myelin content in peripheral nerve? Magn Reson Med 2003;49(4):638–45.

52. Gareau PJ, Rutt BK, Karlik SJ, et al. Magnetization transfer and multicomponent T2 relaxation measurements with histopathologic correlation in an experimental model of MS. J Magn Reson Imaging 2000;11(6):586–95.

53. Beaulieu C, Fenrich FR, Allen PS. Multicomponent water proton transverse relaxation and T2-discriminated water diffusion in myelinated and nonmyelinated nerve. Magn Reson Imaging 1998;16(10):1201–10.

54. Tozer DJ, Davies GR, Altmann DR, et al. Correlation of apparent myelin measures obtained in multiple sclerosis patients and controls from magnetization transfer and multicompartmental T2 analysis. Magn Reson Med 2005;53(6):1415–22.

55. Lawson CL, Hanson RJ. Solving least squares problems. Englewood Cliffs (NJ): Prentice-Hall; 1974.

56. Armspach JP, Gounot D, Rumbach L, et al. In vivo determination of multiexponential T2 relaxation in the brain of patients with multiple sclerosis. Magn Reson Imaging 1991;9(1):107–13.

57. Lancaster JL, Andrews T, Hardies LJ, et al. Three-pool model of white matter. J Magn Reson Imaging 2003;17(1):1–10.

58. Vermathen P, Robert-Tissot L, Pietz J, et al. Characterization of white matter alterations in phenylketonuria by magnetic resonance relaxometry and diffusion tensor imaging. Magn Reson Med 2007;58(6):1145–56.

59. Du YP, Chu R, Hwang D, et al. Fast multislice mapping of the myelin water fraction using multicompartment analysis of T2* decay at 3T: a preliminary postmortem study. Magn Reson Med 2007;58(5):865–70.

60. Deoni SC, Rutt BK, Arun T, et al. Gleaning multi-component T1 and T2 information from steady-state imaging data. Presented at the 16th Annual Meeting of the International Society for Magnetic Resonance in Medicine. Toronto, Canada, 2008.

61. Frahm J, Merboldt KD, Hanicke W. Direct FLASH MR imaging of magnetic field inhomogeneities by gradient compensation. Magn Reson Med 1988; 6(4):474–80.

62. Fernandez-Seara MA, Wehrli FW. Postprocessing technique to correct for background gradients in image-based R*(2) measurements. Magn Reson Med 2000;44(3):358–66.

63. Dahnke H, Schaeffter T. Limits of detection of SPIO at 3.0 T using T2 relaxometry. Magn Reson Med 2005;53(5):1202–6.

64. Kiselev VG. Effect of magnetic field gradients induced by vasculature on NMR measurements of molecular self-diffusion in biological tissues. J Magn Reson 2004;170(2):228–35.

65. Yablonskiy DA. Quantitation of intrinsic magnetic susceptibility-related effects in a tissue matrix: phantom study. Magn Reson Med 1998;39(3):417–28.

66. Conturo TE, Smith GD. Signal-to-noise in phase angle reconstruction: dynamic range extension using phase reference offsets. Magn Reson Med 1990; 15(3):420–37.

67. Witoszynskyj S, Rauscher A, Reichenbach JR, et al. Phase unwrapping of MR images using [Phi]UN – A fast and robust region growing algorithm. Medical Image Analysis, in press.

68. Rauscher A, Barth M, Reichenbach JR, et al. Automated unwrapping of MR phase images applied to BOLD MR-venography at 3 Tesla. J Magn Reson Imaging 2003;18(2):175–80.

69. Jenkinson M, Bannister P, Brady M, et al. Improved optimization for the robust and accurate linear registration and motion correction of brain images. Neuroimage 2002;17(2):825–41.

70. Chavez S, Xiang QS, An L. Understanding phase maps in MRI: a new cutline phase unwrapping method. IEEE Trans Med Imaging 2002;21(8): 966–77.

71. Kamman RL, Go KG, Brouwer W, et al. Nuclear magnetic resonance relaxation in experimental brain edema: effects of water concentration, protein concentration, and temperature. Magn Reson Med 1988;6(3):265–74.

72. Fatouros PP, Marmarou A. Experimental studies for use of magnetic resonance in brain water measurements. Acta Neurochir Suppl 1990;51: 37–8.

73. Fatouros PP, Marmarou A, Kraft KA, et al. In vivo brain water determination by T1 measurements: effect of total water content, hydration fraction, and field strength. Magn Reson Med 1991;17(2):402–13.

74. Kamman RL, Go KG, Stomp GP, et al. Changes of relaxation times T1 and T2 in rat tissues after biopsy and fixation. Magn Reson Imaging 1985; 3(3):245–50.

75. MacDonald HL, Bell BA, Smith MA, et al. Correlation of human NMR T1 values measured in vivo and brain water content. Br J Radiol 1986; 59(700):355–7.

76. Koenig SH, Brown RD 3rd, Spiller M, et al. Relaxometry of brain: why white matter appears bright in MRI. Magn Reson Med 1990;14(3):482–95.

77. Fatouros PP, Marmarou A. Use of magnetic resonance imaging for in vivo measurements of water content in human brain: method and normal values. J Neurosurg 1999;90(1):109–15.

78. Naruse S, Horikawa Y, Tanaka C, et al. Significance of proton relaxation time measurement in brain oedema, cerebral infarction and brain tumors. Magn Reson Med 1986;4:293–304.

79. Rooney WD, Johnson G, Li X, et al. Magnetic field and tissue dependencies of human brain longitudinal 1H2O relaxation in vivo. Magn Reson Med 2007;57(2):308–18.

80. Gelman N, Ewing JR, Gorell JM, et al. Interregional variation of longitudinal relaxation rates in human brain at 3.0 T: relation to estimated iron and water contents. Magn Reson Med 2001;45(1):71–9.

81. Prantner A, Bretthorst G, Neil J, et al. Tissue (brain) water longitudinal relaxation is biexponential. Presented at the 16th Annual Meeting of the International Society for Magnetic Resonance in Medicine. Toronto, Canada, 2008.

82. Labadie C, Lee J-H, Jarchow S, et al. Detection of the myelin water fraction in 4 Tesla longitudinal relaxation data by cross-regularised inverse Laplace transform. Presented at the 16th Annual Meeting of the International Society for Magnetic Resonance in Medicine. Toronto, Canada, 2008.

83. Tofts PS, editor. Quantitative MRI of the brain: measuring changes caused by disease. Chichester West Sussex: Wiley; 2003. p. 316.

84. Swift TJ, Fritz OG Jr. A proton spin-echo study of the state of water in frog nerves. Biophys J 1969;9(1):54–9.

85. Vasilescu V, Katona E, Simplaceanu V, et al. Water compartments in the myelinated nerve. III. Pulsed NMR results. Experientia 1978;34(11):1443–4.

86. Menon RS, Allen PS. Application of continuous relaxation time distributions to the fitting of data from model systems and excised tissue. Magn Reson Med 1991;20(2):214–27.

87. Does MD, Snyder RE. T2 relaxation of peripheral nerve measured in vivo. Magn Reson Imaging 1995;13(4):575–80.

88. MacKay A, Whittall K, Adler J, et al. In vivo visualization of myelin water in brain by magnetic resonance. Magn Reson Med 1994;31(6):673–7.

89. Laule C, Leung E, Lis DK, et al. Myelin water imaging in multiple sclerosis: quantitative correlations with histopathology. Mult Scler 2006;12(6):747–53.

90. Laule C, Kozlowski P, Leung E, et al. Myelin water imaging of multiple sclerosis at 7 T: correlations with histopathology. Neuroimage 2008;40:1575–80.

91. Wu Y, Alexander AL, Fleming JO, et al. Myelin water fraction in human cervical spinal cord in vivo. J Comput Assist Tomogr 2006;30(2):304–6.

92. Minty E, MacKay A, Whittall KP. Measurement of myelin water in human and bovine spinal cord. Presented at the 10th Annual Meeting of the International Society of Magnetic Resonance in Medicine. Honolulu, HI, 2002.

93. Laule C, Vavasour IM, Vavasour JD, et al. Cervical cord abnormalities in primary progressive multiple sclerosis: atrophy and myelin water changes. Presented at the 12th Meeting of the International Society of Magnetic Resonance in Medicine. Kyoto, Japan, 2004.

94. MacMillan EL, Curt A, Maedler B, et al. 3D myelin water imaging of cervical spondylotic myelopathy at 3T. Presented at the 16th Annual Meeting of the International Society for Magnetic Resonance in Medicine. Toronto, Canada, 2008.

95. Jones CK, Xiang QS, Whittall KP, et al. Linear combination of multiecho data: short T2 component selection. Magn Reson Med 2004;51(3):495–502.

96. Vidarsson L, Conolly SM, Lim KO, et al. Echo time optimization for linear combination myelin imaging. Magn Reson Med 2005;53(2):398–407.

97. Stanisz GJ, Kecojevic A, Bronskill MJ, et al. Characterizing white matter with magnetization transfer and T(2). Magn Reson Med 1999;42(6):1128–36.

98. Harrison R, Bronskill MJ, Henkelman RM. Magnetization transfer and T2 relaxation components in tissue. Magn Reson Med 1995;33(4):490–6.

99. Peters AM, Brookes MJ, Hoogenraad FG, et al. T2* measurements in human brain at 1.5, 3 and 7 T. Magn Reson Imaging 2007;25(6):748–53.

100. Silvennoinen MJ, Clingman CS, Golay X, et al. Comparison of the dependence of blood R2 and R2* on oxygen saturation at 1.5 and 4.7 Tesla. Magn Reson Med 2003;49(1):47–60.

101. Zhao JM, Clingman CS, Narvainen MJ, et al. Oxygenation and hematocrit dependence of transverse relaxation rates of blood at 3T. Magn Reson Med 2007;58(3):592–7.

102. Koopmans PJ, Manniesing R, Niessen WJ, et al. MR venography of the human brain using susceptibility weighted imaging at very high field strength. MAGMA 2008;21(1–2):149–58.

103. Norris DG. Principles of magnetic resonance assessment of brain function. J Magn Reson Imaging 2006;23(6):794–807.

104. Meindl T, Born C, Britsch S, et al. Functional BOLD MRI: comparison of different field strengths in a motor task. Eur Radiol 2008;18(6):1102–13.

105. Reichenbach JR, Essig M, Haacke EM, et al. High-resolution venography of the brain using magnetic resonance imaging. MAGMA 1998;6(1):62–9.

106. Haacke EM, Xu Y, Cheng YC, et al. Susceptibility weighted imaging (SWI). Magn Reson Med 2004; 52(3):612–8.

107. Xu Y, Haacke EM. The role of voxel aspect ratio in determining apparent vascular phase behavior in susceptibility weighted imaging. Magn Reson Imaging 2006;24(2):155–60.

108. Lin W, Mukherjee P, An H, et al. Improving high-resolution MR bold venographic imaging using a T1 reducing contrast agent. J Magn Reson Imaging 1999;10(2):118–23.

109. Reichenbach JR, Barth M, Haacke EM, et al. High-resolution MR venography at 3.0 Tesla. J Comput Assist Tomogr 2000;24(6):949–57.

110. Hoogenraad FG, Reichenbach JR, Haacke EM, et al. In vivo measurement of changes in venous blood-oxygenation with high resolution functional MRI at 0.95 Tesla by measuring changes in susceptibility and velocity. Magn Reson Med 1998; 39(1):97–107.

111. Barth M, Reichenbach JR, Venkatesan R, et al. High-resolution, multiple gradient-echo functional MRI at 1.5 T. Magn Reson Imaging 1999;17(3):321–9.

112. Barth M, Norris DG. Very high-resolution three-dimensional functional MRI of the human visual cortex with elimination of large venous vessels. NMR Biomed 2007;20(5):477–84.

113. Young IR, Khenia S, Thomas DG, et al. Clinical magnetic susceptibility mapping of the brain. J Comput Assist Tomogr 1987;11(1):2–6.

114. Yamada N, Imakita S, Sakuma T, et al. Evaluation of the susceptibility effect on the phase images of a simple gradient echo. Radiology 1990;175(2): 561–5.

115. Rauscher A, Sedlacik J, Barth M, et al. Magnetic susceptibility-weighted MR phase imaging of the human brain. AJNR Am J Neuroradiol 2005;26(4): 736–42.

116. Deistung A, Mentzel H-J, Rauscher A, et al. Demonstration of paramagnetic and diamagnetic cerebral lesions by using susceptibility weighted phase imaging (SWI). Z Med Phys 2006;16(4):261–7.

117. Deistung A, Rauscher A, Sedlacik J, et al. Informatics in radiology. GUIBOLD: a graphical user interface for image reconstruction and data analysis in susceptibility-weighted MR imaging. Radiographics 2008;28(3):639–51.

118. Duyn JH, van Gelderen P, Li T-Q, et al. High-field MRI of brain cortical substructure based on signal phase. Proc Natl Acad Sci USA 2007;104(28): 11796–801.

119. Ogg RJ, Langston JW, Haacke EM, et al. The cor-relation between phase shifts in gradient-echo MR images and regional brain iron concentration. Magn Reson Imaging 1999;17(8):1141–8.

120. Hallgren B, Sourander P. The effect of age on the non-haemin iron in the human brain. J Neurochem 1958;3:41–51.

121. Haacke EM, Ayaz M, Khan A, et al. Establishing a baseline phase behavior in magnetic resonance imaging to determine normal vs. abnormal iron content in the brain. J Magn Reson Imaging 2007;26(2):256–64.

122. Xu X, Wang Q, Zhang M. Age, gender, and hemi-spheric differences in iron deposition in the human brain: an in vivo MRI study. Neuroimage 2008; 40(1):35–42.

123. Zhong K, Leupold J, von Elverfeldt D, et al. The molecular basis for gray and white matter contrast in phase imaging. Neuroimage 2008;40(4):1561–6.

124. Ormerod IEC, Bronstein A, Rudge P, et al. Mag-netic resonance imaging in clinically isolated le-sions of the brain stem. J Neurol Neurosurg Psychiatry 1986;49:737–43.

125. Larsson HB, Frederiksen J, Petersen J, et al. Assessment of demyelination, edema, and gliosis by in vivo determination of T1 and T2 in the brain of patients with acute attack of multiple sclerosis. Magn Reson Med 1989;11(3):337–48.

126. Larsson HB, Frederiksen J, Kjaer L, et al. In vivo determination of T1 and T2 in the brain of patients with severe but stable multiple sclerosis. Magn Reson Med 1988;7(1):43–55.

127. Vavasour IM, Li DK, Laule C, et al. Multi-parametric MR assessment of T(1) black holes in multiple scle-rosis: evidence that myelin loss is not greater in hy-pointense versus isointense T(1) lesions. J Neurol 2007;254(12):1653–9.

128. Vavasour IM, Li DKB, Laule C, et al. Myelin water is an independent measure of pathology in multiple sclerosis. Presented at ISMRM. Seattle, WA, 2006.

129. Stevenson VL, Parker GJ, Barker GJ, et al. Varia-tions in T1 and T2 relaxation times of normal appearing white matter and lesions in multiple scle-rosis. J Neurol Sci. 2000;178(2):81–7.

130. Truyen L, van Waesberghe JH, van Walderveen MA, et al. Accumulation of hypoin-tense lesions ("black holes") on T1 spin-echo MRI correlates with disease progression in multiple sclerosis. Neurology 1996;47(6):1469–76.

131. McDonald WI, Miller DH, Thompson AJ. Are mag-netic resonance findings predictive of clinical out-come in therapeutic trials in multiple sclerosis? The dilemma of interferon-beta. Ann Neurol 1994; 36(1):14–8.

132. Miki Y, Grossman RI, Udupa JK, et al. Relapsing-remitting multiple sclerosis: longitudinal analysis of MR images. Lack of correlation between changes in T2 lesion volume and clinical findings. Radiology 1999;213(2):395–9.

133. van Walderveen MA, Barkhof F, Hommes OR, et al. Correlating MRI and clinical disease activity in mul-tiple sclerosis: relevance of hypointense lesions on short-TR/short-TE (T1-weighted) spin-echo im-ages. Neurology 1995;45(9):1684–90.

134. Cid C, Alcazar A, Regidor I, et al. Neuronal apopto-sis induced by cerebrospinal fluid from multiple sclerosis patients correlates with hypointense le-sions on T1 magnetic resonance imaging. J Neurol Sci 2002;193(2):103–9.

135. Sailer M, Losseff NA, Wang L, et al. T1 lesion load and cerebral atrophy as a marker for clinical pro-gression in patients with multiple sclerosis: a pro-spective 18 months follow-up study. Eur J Neurol 2001;8(1):37–42.

136. Simon JH, Lull J, Jacobs LD, et al. Multiple Sclero-sis Collaborative Research Group. A longitudinal study of T1 hypointense lesions in relapsing MS: MSCRG trial of interferon beta-1a. Neurology 2000;55(2):185–92.

137. van Walderveen MA, Lycklama ANGJ, Ader HJ, et al. Hypointense lesions on T1-weighted spin-echo magnetic resonance imaging: relation to clinical characteristics in subgroups of patients with multiple sclerosis. Arch Neurol 2001;58(1): 76–81.

138. Bagnato F, Jeffries N, Richert ND, et al. Evolution of T1 black holes in patients with multiple sclerosis imaged monthly for 4 years. Brain 2003;126(Pt 8): 1782–9.

139. van Walderveen MA, Barkhof F, Pouwels PJ, et al. Neuronal damage in T1-hypointense multiple scle-rosis lesions demonstrated in vivo using proton magnetic resonance spectroscopy. Ann Neurol 1999;46(1):79–87.

140. Li BS, Regal J, Soher BJ, et al. Brain metabolite profiles of T1-hypointense lesions in relapsing-re-mitting multiple sclerosis. AJNR Am J Neuroradiol 2003;24(1):68–74.

141. Nusbaum AO, Lu D, Tang CY, et al. Quantitative dif-fusion measurements in focal multiple sclerosis le-sions: correlations with appearance on TI-weighted MR images. AJR Am J Roentgenol 2000;175(3): 821–5.

142. Nusbaum AO, Tang CY, Wei TC, et al. Whole-brain diffusion MR histograms differ between MS sub-types. Neurology 2000;54(7):1421–7.

143. Droogan AG, Clark CA, Werring DJ, et al. Compar-ison of multiple sclerosis clinical subgroups using navigated spin echo diffusion-weighted imaging. Magn Reson Imaging 1999;17(5):653–61.

144. Castriota-Scanderbeg A, Fasano F, Hagberg G, et al. Coefficient D(av) is more sensitive than frac-tional anisotropy in monitoring progression of irre-versible tissue damage in focal nonactive multiple

sclerosis lesions. AJNR Am J Neuroradiol 2003; 24(4):663–70.

145. Brück W, Bitsch A, Kolenda H, et al. Inflammatory central nervous system demyelination: correlation of magnetic resonance imaging findings with lesion pathology. Ann Neurol 1997;42(5):783–93.

146. van Walderveen MA, Kamphorst W, Scheltens P, et al. Histopathologic correlate of hypointense lesions on T1-weighted spin-echo MRI in multiple sclerosis. Neurology 1998;50(5):1282–8.

147. van Waesberghe JH, Kamphorst W, De Groot CJ, et al. Axonal loss in multiple sclerosis lesions: magnetic resonance imaging insights into substrates of disability. Ann Neurol 1999;46(5):747–54.

148. Bitsch A, Kuhlmann T, Stadelmann C, et al. A longitudinal MRI study of histopathologically defined hypointense multiple sclerosis lesions. Ann Neurol 2001;49(6):793–6.

149. Haughton VM, Yetkin FZ, Rao SM, et al. Quantitative MR in the diagnosis of multiple sclerosis. Magn Reson Med 1992;26(1):71–8.

150. Miller DH, Johnson G, Tofts PS, et al. Precise relaxation time measurements of normal-appearing white matter in inflammatory central nervous system disease. Magn Reson Med 1989;11(3):331–6.

151. Brainin M, Neuhold A, Reisner T, et al. Changes within the "normal" cerebral white matter of multiple sclerosis patients during acute attacks and during high-dose cortisone therapy assessed by means of quantitative MRI. J Neurol Neurosurg Psychiatr 1989;52(12):1355–9.

152. Lacomis D, Osbakken M, Gross G. Spin-lattice relaxation (T1) times of cerebral white matter in multiple sclerosis. Magn Reson Med 1986;3(2):194–202.

153. Kesselring J, Miller DH, MacManus DG, et al. Quantitative magnetic resonance imaging in multiple sclerosis: the effect of high dose intravenous methylprednisolone. J Neurol Neurosurg Psychiatr 1989;52(1):14–7.

154. Barbosa S, Blumhardt LD, Roberts N, et al. Magnetic resonance relaxation time mapping in multiple sclerosis: normal appearing white matter and the "invisible" lesion load. Magn Reson Imaging 1994;12(1):33–42.

155. Castriota-Scanderbeg A, Fasano F, Filippi M, et al. T1 relaxation maps allow differentiation between pathologic tissue subsets in relapsing-remitting and secondary progressive multiple sclerosis. Mult Scler 2004;10(5):556–61.

156. Davies GR, Hadjiprocopis A, Altmann DR, et al. Normal-appearing grey and white matter T1 abnormality in early relapsing-remitting multiple sclerosis: a longitudinal study. Mult Scler 2007;13(2):169–77.

157. Parry A, Clare S, Jenkinson M, et al. White matter and lesion T1 relaxation times increase in parallel and correlate with disability in multiple sclerosis. J Neurol 2002;249(9):1279–86.

158. Srinivasan R, Henry R, Pelletier D, et al. Standardized, reproducible, high resolution global measurements of T1 relaxation metrics in cases of multiple sclerosis. AJNR Am J Neuroradiol 2003;24(1):58–67.

159. Vrenken H, Geurts JJ, Knol DL, et al. Whole-brain T1 mapping in multiple sclerosis: global changes of normal-appearing gray and white matter. Radiology 2006;240(3):811–20.

160. Vrenken H, Rombouts SA, Pouwels PJ, et al. Voxel-based analysis of quantitative T1 maps demonstrates that multiple sclerosis acts throughout the normal-appearing white matter. AJNR Am J Neuroradiol 2006;27(4):868–74.

161. Barkhof F. Whole-brain T1-relaxation time measurements in multiple sclerosis. J Neurol 2002;249(10):1451–2.

162. van Walderveen MA, van Schijndel RA, Pouwels PJ, et al. Multislice T1 relaxation time measurements in the brain using IR-EPI: reproducibility, normal values, and histogram analysis in patients with multiple sclerosis. J Magn Reson Imaging 2003;18(6):656–64.

163. Parry A, Clare S, Jenkinson M, et al. MRI brain T1 relaxation time changes in MS patients increase over time in both the white matter and the cortex. J Neuroimaging 2003;13(3):234–9.

164. Manfredonia F, Ciccarelli O, Khaleeli Z, et al. Normal-appearing brain T1 relaxation time predicts disability in early primary progressive multiple sclerosis. Arch Neurol 2007;64(3):411–5.

165. Vrenken H, Geurts JJ, Knol DL, et al. Normal-appearing white matter changes vary with distance to lesions in multiple sclerosis. AJNR Am J Neuroradiol 2006;27(9):2005–11.

166. Vaithianathar L, Tench CR, Morgan PS, et al. T1 relaxation time mapping of white matter tracts in multiple sclerosis defined by diffusion tensor imaging. J Neurol 2002;249(9):1272–8.

167. Vaithianathar L, Tench CR, Morgan PS, et al. White matter T(1) relaxation time histograms and cerebral atrophy in multiple sclerosis. J Neurol Sci 2002;197(1-2):45–50.

168. Brex PA, Parker GJ, Leary SM, et al. Lesion heterogeneity in multiple sclerosis: a study of the relations between appearances on T1 weighted images, T1 relaxation times, and metabolite concentrations. J Neurol Neurosurg Psychiatr 2000;68(5):627–32.

169. Vaithianathar L, Tench CR, Morgan PS, et al. Magnetic resonance imaging of the cervical spinal cord in multiple sclerosis—a quantitative T1 relaxation time mapping approach. J Neurol 2003;250(3):307–15.

170. Mottershead JP, Schmierer K, Clemence M, et al. High field MRI correlates of myelin content and axonal density in multiple sclerosis: a post-mortem

study of the spinal cord. J Neurol 2003;250(11): 1293–301.

171. Goodkin DE, Rooney WD, Sloan R, et al. A serial study of new MS lesions and the white matter from which they arise. Neurology 1998;51(6):1689–97.

172. Vavasour IM, MacKay AL, Whittall KP, et al. A serial magnetic resonance study of multiple sclerosis: T2 relaxation, T1 relaxation and magnetization transfer. Presented at the 51st Annual Meeting of the American Academy of Neurology. Toronto, Canada, 1999.

173. Barnes D, Munro PM, Youl BD, et al. The long-standing MS lesion: a quantitative MRI and electron microscopic study. Brain 1991;114(Pt 3): 1271–80.

174. Papanikolaou N, Papadaki E, Karampekios S, et al. T2 relaxation time analysis in patients with multiple sclerosis: correlation with magnetization transfer ratio. Eur Radiol 2004;14(1):115–22.

175. Filippi M, Barker GJ, Horsfield MA, et al. Benign and secondary progressive multiple sclerosis: a preliminary quantitative MRI study. J Neurol 1994;241:246–51.

176. Kidd D, Barker GJ, Tofts PS, et al. The transverse magnetisation decay characteristics of longstanding lesions and normal-appearing white matter in multiple sclerosis. J Neurol 1997;244(2):125–30.

177. Laule C, Vavasour IM, Moore GRW, et al. Water content and myelin water fraction in multiple sclerosis: a T2 relaxation study. J Neurol 2004;251(3): 284–93.

178. Oh J, Han ET, Lee MC, et al. Multislice brain myelin water fractions at 3T in multiple sclerosis. J Neuroimaging 2007;17(2):156–63.

179. Whittall KP, MacKay AL, Li DK, et al. Normal-appearing white matter in multiple sclerosis has heterogeneous, diffusely prolonged T(2). Magn Reson Med 2002;47(2):403–8.

180. Grenier D, Pelletier D, Normandeau M, et al. T2 relaxation time histograms in multiple sclerosis. Magn Reson Imaging 2002;20(10):733–41.

181. Filippi M, Rocca MA, Martino G, et al. Magnetization transfer changes in the normal appearing white matter precede the appearance of enhancing lesions in patients with multiple sclerosis. Ann Neurol 1998;43(6):809–14.

182. Pike GB, De Stefano N, Narayanan S, et al. Multiple sclerosis: magnetization transfer MR imaging of white matter before lesion appearance on T2-weighted images. Radiology 2000;215(3):824–30.

183. Richert ND, Ostuni JL, Bash CN, et al. Interferon beta-1b and intravenous methylprednisolone promote lesion recovery in multiple sclerosis. Mult Scler 2001;7(1):49–58.

184. Narayana PA, Doyle TJ, Lai D, et al. Serial proton magnetic resonance spectroscopic imaging, contrast-enhanced magnetic resonance imaging, and quantitative lesion volumetry in multiple sclerosis. Ann Neurol 1998;43(1):56–71.

185. Werring DJ, Brassat D, Droogan AG, et al. The pathogenesis of lesions and normal-appearing white matter changes in multiple sclerosis: a serial diffusion MRI study. Brain 2000;123(Pt 8): 1667–76.

186. Moore GRW, Leung E, MacKay AL, et al. A pathology-MRI study of the short-T2 component in formalin-fixed multiple sclerosis brain. Neurology 2000; 55(10):1506–10.

187. Ramani A, Aliev AE, Barker GJ, et al. Another approach to protons with constricted mobility in white matter: pilot studies using wideline and high-resolution NMR spectroscopy. Magn Reson Imaging 2003;21(9):1039–43.

188. Tan IL, van Schijndel RA, Pouwels PJ, et al. MR venography of multiple sclerosis. AJNR Am J Neuroradiol 2000;21(6):1039–42.

189. Dixon J, Tallantyre E, Morgan PS, et al. Susceptibility-weighted MR imaging of vascular distribution in white-matter MS lesions. Presented at the 16th Annual Meeting of the International Society for Magnetic Resonance in Medicine. Toronto, Canada, 2008.

190. Haacke EM, Makki M, Ge Y, et al. Correlating iron with T2 signal intensity in multiple sclerosis lesions using susceptibility weighted imaging. Presented at the16th Annual Meeting of the International Society for Magnetic Resonance in Medicine. Toronto, Canada, 2008.

191. Eissa A, Lebel R, Korzan J, et al. MRI of multiple sclerosis with high contrast susceptibility-weighting and extreme resolution T2-weighting. Presented at the 16th Annual Meeting of the International Society for Magnetic Resonance in Medicine. Toronto, Canada, 2008.

192. Hammond KE, Lupo JM, Xu D, et al. Development of a robust method for generating 7.0 T multichannel phase images of the brain with application to normal volunteers and patients with neurological diseases. Neuroimage 2008;39(4):1682–92.

193. Shah J, Rammohan K, Racke M, et al. New approaches for ms lesion characterization with ultrahigh field MSRI: comparison of T2*/phase susceptibility weighted images with T2- and inversion recovery fast spin echo sequences. Presented at the16th Annual Meeting of the International Society for Magnetic Resonance in Medicine. Toronto, Canada, 2008.

194. Pantano P, Mainero C, Caramia F. Functional brain reorganization in multiple sclerosis: evidence from fMRI studies. J Neuroimaging 2006;16(2):104–14.

195. Buckle GJ. Functional magnetic resonance imaging and multiple sclerosis: the evidence for neuronal plasticity. J Neuroimaging 2005;15(4 Suppl): 82s–93s.

196. Rocca MA, Filippi M. Functional MRI in multiple sclerosis. J Neuroimaging 2007;17(Suppl 1):36s–41s.

197. Strijkers GJ, Mulder WJ, van Tilborg GA, et al. MRI contrast agents: current status and future perspectives. Anticancer Agents Med Chem 2007; 7(3):291–305.

198. Sibson NR, Blamire AM, Bernades-Silva M, et al. MRI detection of early endothelial activation in brain inflammation. Magn Reson Med 2004;51(2):248–52.

199. Wessig C, Bendszus M, Stoll G. In vivo visualization of focal demyelination in peripheral nerves by gadofluorine M-enhanced magnetic resonance imaging. Exp Neurol 2007;204(1):14–9.

200. Vellinga MM, Oude Engberink RD, Seewann A, et al. Pluriformity of inflammation in multiple sclerosis shown by ultra-small iron oxide particle enhancement. Brain 2008;131(Pt 3):800–7.

201. Dousset V, Brochet B, Deloire MS, et al. MR imaging of relapsing multiple sclerosis patients using ultra-small-particle iron oxide and compared with gadolinium. AJNR Am J Neuroradiol 2006;27(5):1000–5.

202. Oweida AJ, Dunn EA, Karlik SJ, et al. Iron-oxide labeling of hematogenous macrophages in a model of experimental autoimmune encephalomyelitis and the contribution to signal loss in fast imaging employing steady state acquisition (FIESTA) images. J Magn Reson Imaging 2007;26(1):144–51.

203. Brochet B, Deloire MS, Touil T, et al. Early macrophage MRI of inflammatory lesions predicts lesion severity and disease development in relapsing EAE. Neuroimage 2006;32(1):266–74.

204. Heyn C, Ronald JA, Mackenzie LT, et al. In vivo magnetic resonance imaging of single cells in mouse brain with optical validation. Magn Reson Med 2006;55(1):23–9.

205. Anderson SA, Shukaliak-Quandt J, Jordan EK, et al. Magnetic resonance imaging of labeled T-cells in a mouse model of multiple sclerosis. Ann Neurol 2004;55(5):654–9.

206. Frank JA, Miller BR, Arbab AS, et al. Clinically applicable labeling of mammalian and stem cells by combining superparamagnetic iron oxides and transfection agents. Radiology 2003;228(2):480–7.

207. Moseley ME, Cohen Y, Kucharczyk J, et al. Diffusion-weighted MR imaging of anisotropic water diffusion in cat central nervous system. Radiology 1990;176(2):439–45.

208. Thomsen C, Henriksen O, Ring P. In vivo measurement of water self diffusion in the human brain by magnetic resonance imaging. Acta Radiol 1987; 28(3):353–61.

209. Basser PJ. Inferring structural features and the physiological state of tissues from diffusion-weighted images. NMR Biomed 1995;8(7–8):333–44.

210. Basser PJ, Pajevic S. Statistical artifacts in diffusion tensor MRI (DT-MRI) caused by background noise. Magn Reson Med 2000;44(1):41–50.

211. Xue R, van Zijl PCM, Crain BJ, et al. In vivo three-dimensional reconstruction of rat brain axonal projections by diffusion tensor imaging. Magn Reson Med 1999;42(6):1123–7.

212. Beaulieu C, Does MD, Snyder RE, et al. Changes in water diffusion due to Wallerian degeneration in peripheral nerve. Magn Reson Med 1996;36(4): 627–31.

213. Biton IE, Duncan ID, Cohen Y. High b-value q-space diffusion MRI in myelin-deficient rat spinal cords. Magn Reson Imaging 2006;24(2):161–6 Epub 2005 Dec 2027.

214. Kim JH, Budde MD, Liang HF, et al. Detecting axon damage in spinal cord from a mouse model of multiple sclerosis. Neurobiol Dis 2006;21(3):626–32 Epub 2005 Nov 2017.

215. Song SK, Sun SW, Ju WK, et al. Diffusion tensor imaging detects and differentiates axon and myelin degeneration in mouse optic nerve after retinal ischemia. Neuroimage 2003;20(3):1714–22.

216. Song SK, Sun SW, Ramsbottom MJ, et al. Dysmyelination revealed through MRI as increased radial (but unchanged axial) diffusion of water. Neuroimage 2002;17(3):1429–36.

217. Song SK, Yoshino J, Le TQ, et al. Demyelination increases radial diffusivity in corpus callosum of mouse brain. Neuroimage 2005;26(1):132–40.

218. Sun SW, Liang HF, Le TQ, et al. Differential sensitivity of in vivo and ex vivo diffusion tensor imaging to evolving optic nerve injury in mice with retinal ischemia. Neuroimage 2006;32(3):1195–204. Epub 2006 Jun 1122.

219. Sun SW, Liang HF, Trinkaus K, et al. Noninvasive detection of cuprizone induced axonal damage and demyelination in the mouse corpus callosum. Magn Reson Med 2006;55(2):302–8.

220. Thomalla G, Glauche V, Koch MA, et al. Diffusion tensor imaging detects early Wallerian degeneration of the pyramidal tract after ischemic stroke. Neuroimage 2004;22(4):1767–74.

221. Mädler B, Drabycz SA, Kolind SH, et al. Is diffusion anisotropy an accurate monitor of myelination? Correlation of multicomponent T2 relaxation and diffusion tensor anisotropy in human brain. Magn Reson Imaging 2008;26(7):874–88.

222. Bells S, Morris D, Vidarsson L. Comparison of linear combination filtering to DTI and MTR in whole brain myelin-water imaging. Presented at the 15th Annual Meeting of the International Society of Magnetic Resonance in Medicine. Berlin, Germany, 2007.

223. Beaulieu C. The basis of anisotropic water diffusion in the nervous system: a technical review. NMR Biomed 2002;15(7–8):435–55.

224. Kolind SH, Laule C, Vavasour IM, et al. Complementary information from multi-exponential T(2) relaxation and diffusion tensor imaging reveals

differences between multiple sclerosis lesions. Neuroimage 2008;40(1):77–85.

225. Tyszka JM, Readhead C, Bearer EL, et al. Statistical diffusion tensor histology reveals regional dysmyelination effects in the shiverer mouse mutant. Neuroimage 2006;29(4):1058–65.

226. Wu Y-C, Alexander AL, Duncan ID, et al. Hybrid diffusion imaging in a brain model of dysmyelination. Presented at the 15th Annual Meeting of the International Society of Magnetic Resonance in Medicine. Berlin, Germany, 2007.

227. van Waesberghe JH, Castelijns JA, Scheltens P, et al. Comparison of four potential MR parameters for severe tissue destruction in multiple sclerosis lesions. Magn Reson Imaging 1997;15(2):155–62.

228. Griffin CM, Parker GJ, Barker GJ, et al. MTR and T1 provide complementary information in MS NAWM, but not in lesions. Mult Scler 2000;6(5):327–31.

229. Schmierer K, Scaravilli F, Altmann DR, et al. Magnetization transfer ratio and myelin in postmortem multiple sclerosis brain. Ann Neurol 2004;56(3):407–15.

230. Karampekios S, Papanikolaou N, Papadaki E, et al. Quantification of magnetization transfer rate and native T1 relaxation time of the brain: correlation with magnetization transfer ratio measurements in patients with multiple sclerosis. Neuroradiology 2005;47(3):189–96.

231. Vavasour IM. Magnetic resonance of human and bovine brain [doctoral thesis]. Vancouver: University of British Columbia; 1998.

232. Papanikolaou N, Maniatis V, Pappas J, et al. Biexponential T2 relaxation time analysis of the brain: correlation with magnetization transfer ratio. Invest Radiol 2002;37(7):363–7.

233. Wu Y, Field A, Alexander A, et al. Quantification of myelin water in human cervical spinal cord in vivo. Presented at the 12th Annual Meeting of the International Society for Magnetic Resonance in Medicine. Kyoto, Japan, 2004.

234. Helms G, Piringer A. Magnetization transfer of water T(2) relaxation components in human brain: implications for T(2)-based segmentation of spectroscopic volumes. Magn Reson Imaging 2001;19(6):803–11.

235. Morrissey SP, Stodal H, Zettl U, et al. In vivo MRI and its histological correlates in acute adoptive transfer experimental allergic encephalomyelitis: quantification of inflammation and oedema. Brain 1996;119(Pt 1):239–48.

Magnetization Transfer MR Imaging in Multiple Sclerosis

Stefan Ropele, PhD*, Franz Fazekas, MD

KEYWORDS

- Magnetization transfer • Quantitative MRI • Brain
- Multiple sclerosis • White mattter • Myelin

Signal intensities derived by conventional MR imaging are mainly based on the different relaxation characteristics of ^1H protons in water molecules. The tissue-specific microstructure surrounding these water molecules determines the respective relaxation behavior and hence their intrinsic T_1 and T_2 relaxation times. This is the basis for the excellent tissue contrast that has made MR imaging an invaluable tool for the diagnosis and management of disorders of the central nervous system (CNS) and especially of white matter (WM) diseases.

Magnetization transfer (MT) MR imaging is an approach to explore nonwater components in tissue. Protons bound to larger molecules have relaxation properties that make them invisible for a conventional MR measurement. However, the pool of bound protons can be indirectly quantified by MR imaging sequences that use the mechanism of energy exchange between bound protons and water protons, commonly termed MT, and observe the modulation of energy of tissue water protons that results from this process. As the extent of MT largely depends on the structure and biochemical environment of the macromolecules, MT MR imaging thus provides a new and different window into tissue composition and microstructure. The attraction of using MT for assessing tissue changes in multiple sclerosis (MS) is obvious. While conventional MR imaging lacks specificity, MT MR imaging is expected to add independent and quantitative microstructural information on MS-related tissue changes. This is the reason why MT MR imaging has been widely applied in MS research over the past years.

MR sequences for generating MT contrast (MTC) are readily available on modern scanners. MT MR imaging is a robust technique with high reproducibility. The absolute MTC, however, largely depends on sequence and scanner characteristics. Thus, the choice of MT sequence parameters has a huge impact on the magnitude of MTC observed and the resulting sensitivity for the detection of tissue changes. This dependence may be well used for maximizing the MTC but also goes along with the inherent problem of potentially significant variations in the MTC generated with different scanners and at different sites. As a consequence, reported absolute values per se may be insufficient or even misleading when attempting to interpret the results of MT studies and the performance of multicenter studies can be challenging. After introducing fundamental aspects of MT, of MT MR imaging, and the respective analysis techniques we review the applications of this technique to MS and its contribution to our understanding of the disease.

THE PHENOMENON OF MAGNETIZATION TRANSFER

The two-pool model traditionally serves as a simplified model for understanding the phenomenon of MT. Brain tissue is commonly considered as a system with two different kinds of ^1H protons.[1–4] One pool represents the protons of the free mobile tissue water, whereas the other represents motional restricted ^1H protons that are bound to macromolecules. In the case of brain tissue the bound protons are mainly associated with the

Department of Neurology, Medical University Graz, Auenbruggerplatz 22, A-8036 Graz, Austria/Europe.
* Corresponding author.
E-mail address: stefan.ropele@meduni-graz.at (S. Ropele).

Neuroimag Clin N Am 19 (2009) 27–36
doi:10.1016/j.nic.2008.09.004
1052-5149/08/$ – see front matter © 2008 Elsevier Inc. All rights reserved.

myelin lipids and proteins (**Fig. 1**). Compartmentalization of ^{1}H spins in terms of their mobility can also be demonstrated in the frequency domain, where bulk water exhibits a very narrow line width while the signal of the motional restricted ^{1}H protons is significantly broadened. This is also the reason why protons bound to macromolecules are not observable with conventional MR imaging. Recent studies have extended the two-pool model by separating the liquid pool into more dedicated water pools.[5,6] Although the two-pool model is sufficient to describe longitudinal relaxation in brain tissue,[7] the extended model may be particularly important for a T_2 relaxation analysis.[5,8,9]

The most important feature of the two-pool model is the exchange of magnetization between both pools. The amount of MT is usually expressed by a fundamental rate constant or, depending on notation, by a first-order forward and backward transfer rate.

Two different models are currently used to explain the mechanisms of MT between water and protons of macromolecules. Both are based on the nuclear Overhauser effect (NOE), which provides dipole-dipole coupling over very short distances only. One model is based on the assumption that the nonexchangeable protons of macromolecules exchange magnetization with the water protons of the hydration layer by NOE cross relaxation, where hydration water exchanges rapidly with free mobile tissue water. In the other model, exchange of magnetization by NOE cross-relaxation occurs between nonexchangeable protons and exchangeable protons of the NH and OH groups of the macromolecules, which in turn exchange sufficiently fast with tissue water protons (proton exchange). In the latter model no hydration layer is involved in MT.

So far the dominant mechanism in brain tissue that accounts for an efficient MT between water and macromolecules is still unclear. Results from high-resolution MR spectroscopy suggest that the water of the hydration layer has a residence time in the range of subnanoseconds.[10,11] This short residence time is also confirmed by relaxation time measurements of deuteron and ^{17}O spins.[12,13] As a consequence, the hydration water does not appear to stay sufficiently long in contact with the macromolecular surface for a significant contribution to the MT via the NOE. On the other hand, there is evidence that some globular proteins contain internal hydration water molecules that exchange considerably more slowly with the bulk water.[10,13] MT thus is probably restricted to a few sites of the macromolecules, ie, those with relatively long-lived hydration water. Experiments with lipid suspensions and isotopically substituted protons support this view and have shown that the exchange of magnetization is not chemical.[14] Observations of a strong pH effect on MT also suggest the exchange of protons as an important mechanism for MT.[15,16]

In summary, although several potential transfer processes of magnetization have been identified, it is still unclear which one plays the dominant role in the CNS. For the interpretation of MT experiments, knowledge of the exact mechanism involved would certainly be an advantage. In the absence of such an understanding, we currently use to consider MT as a phenomenon that is linked primarily to the density of macromolecules. Furthermore, it is specific for the CNS that the macromolecular density is largely driven by the macromolecules contained in myelin. As a consequence, measurements of MT are especially sensitive to changes in myelination but it is increasingly recognized that the information provided goes far beyond WM.

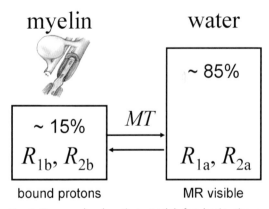

Fig. 1. Two-pool relaxation model for brain tissue. Approximately 15% of ^{1}H protons are bound to the myelin lipids and proteins. MT exchanges their energy with the much larger pool of bulk water. Mathematically, the model can be fully described with the coupled Bloch equations that consider six parameters including the intrinsic relaxation rates (R_1 and R_2), the relative pool sizes, and MT.

IMAGING OF THE MAGNETIZATION TRANSFER

MT MR imaging intends to depict differences in the effect of MT within a given tissue or organ by generating MTC. This is achieved by employing trains of spectral selective radiofrequency (RF) pulses to selectively saturate the longitudinal magnetization of the bound protons, ie, to reduce their magnetization toward zero. This magnetization (or energy) is then "exchanged" with the MR visible water pool ("saturation transfer"), ie, the free water protons also become partly saturated. Consequently, the MR signal intensity that is proportional to the longitudinal magnetization of the water pool goes down (**Fig. 2**). In the two-pool model the amount of signal decrease depends on the rate of exchange, the fractional size of the bound pool, and the intrinsic T_1 and T_2 relaxation times of each pool. Basically, all six pool parameters can be estimated from a series of saturation transfer experiments with varying frequency or power of the saturation pulses.[17–19] However, because of the extensive measurement time that would be necessary and because of complex postprocessing, such an approach is still not feasible in clinical routine. Instead, "conventional" MT measurements assess the relative magnitude of MT, ie, the magnetization transfer ratio (MTR), which can be derived from the combination of a single saturation transfer measurement and a reference measurement. For these measurements, it is desirable to normalize the signal drop caused

by MT, therefore it has become common practice to calculate the MTR according to:

$$MTR = \left(1 - \frac{S_S}{S_0}\right) \cdot 100\%$$

where S_s is the signal intensity obtained under selective saturation and S_0 is a reference measurement without any saturation pulse. The MTR can be calculated for an individual region but also for a whole image by doing this calculation pixelwise (**Fig. 3**).

The MTR has become a very attractive measure because it is sensitive to MT, and it is fast and easy to measure. Moreover, it is a quantitative measure in the sense that it is reproducible and comparable among subjects provided the same sequence is used. However, it is often overlooked that the MTR is generally a weighted function of all pool parameters and therefore strongly depends on the sequence parameters and on the properties of the saturation pulses. This is also the reason why the variation of published MTR values is extremely high.

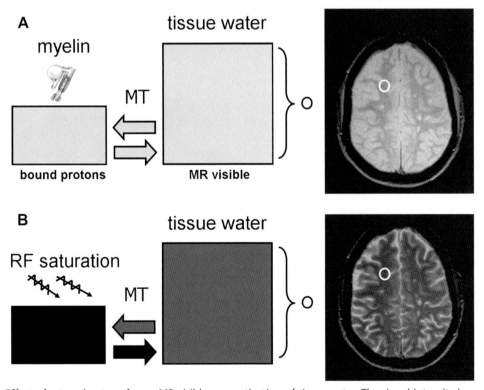

Fig. 2. Effect of saturation transfer on MR visible magnetization of tissue water. The signal intensity in a proton density weighted sequence is proportional to the longitudinal magnetization in the MR visible water pool. Therefore, white matter (WM) appears bright in the reference measurement with no MT saturation (A). Selective RF saturation of the myelin pool results in a significant reduction of the longitudinal magnetization. Because of MT, this saturation is transferred to the MR visible water pool and becomes visible as a signal reduction in areas of high MT, ie, the WM appears darker (B).

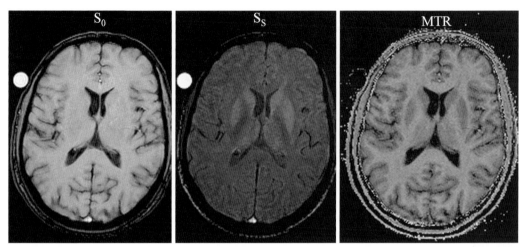

Fig. 3. The MTR can be calculated pixelwise from a reference scan (*left*) and from a scan obtained with MT saturation (*middle*) yielding an MTR map (*right*). The signal intensity in the MTR map reflects the extent of MT, ie, areas with a higher MTR like the WM appear brighter than the cortex, which has a lower MTR. Note that the Gadolineum-doped phantom attached to the head coil provides high signal intensity, but no MT because of the absence of a macromolecular pool.

MTR mapping can be done with almost every pulse sequence just by adding spectral selective saturation pulses. The saturation is usually done with an off-resonance saturation pulse but can also be performed on-resonance. On-resonant pulses consist of a binomial series of rectangular RF pulses. Their saturation effect is comparable with the effect of off-resonance pulses and they are much shorter and therefore more efficient; however, they are also more sensitive to B_0 variations and imperfections of pulse timing.[20–22] MTR mapping is usually done with proton density weighted gradient echo sequences, but also other sequences such as a spin echo sequence or even a true fast imaging with steady state precession (FISP) sequence can be used.[23,24] An interesting option is the use of a gradient echo sequence with a short repetition time.[25,26] This approach allows true three-dimensional imaging and provides a high signal-to-noise ratio in addition to a strong MT saturation effect. The latter is caused by the fact that a shorter repetition time allows more saturation pulses in a given time and therefore a higher rate of RF saturation. It should be noted, however, that in such a setting the signal reduction due to the MT effect can be partly counteracted by T_1 relaxation, ie, MT also reduces T_1, which leads to an increase in signal intensity in T_1-weighted sequences.

Because of the saturation pulses, MT sequences produce a higher power deposition in brain tissue than conventional sequences. While the restriction by the specific absorption rate (SAR) at 1.5 T is usually small for MT sequences, SAR limits hamper the implementation of MT sequences at higher field strength. Therefore, parallel imaging techniques or SAR reduction techniques[27] are required to take advantage of the full benefits provided by high field strengths (**Fig. 4**).

MEASURING MAGNETIZATION TRANSFER RATIO CHANGES

A common approach to assess MTR globally is through histogram analysis (**Fig. 5**). An MTR

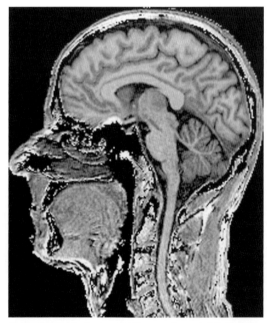

Fig. 4. High-resolution MTR mapping at 3.0 T. Using low SAR techniques, MTR maps with isotropic resolution and high signal-to-noise ratio can be acquired within a few minutes.[27]

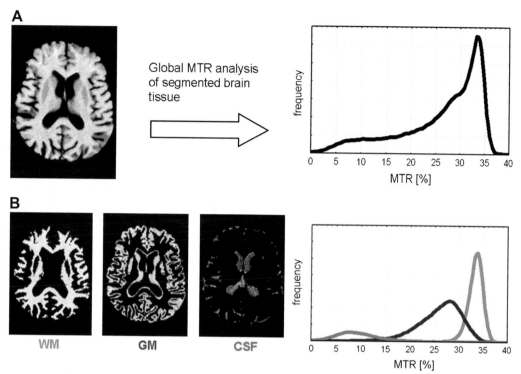

Fig. 5. An MTR histogram from segmented brain tissue (*A*). A histogram from whole brain tissue results from the superimposition of tissue specific MTR peaks, where the most dominant peak stems from the white matter (*B*). CSF exhibits a small MT effect owing to the so-called direct saturation effect, although it contains no macromolecular proton pool.

histogram is a plot of the frequency of each MTR value over a sufficiently large span of MTR values that are observed in a given part of the CNS, eg, a tissue segment, a brain slice, or the entire brain.[28,29] Histograms are usually normalized to correct for different brain sizes and atrophy. At least two essential parameters can be derived from the histogram: the peak position, ie, the MTR value that has been measured most often (with the highest frequency), and the relative height of this peak. As noted above, histograms can be generated for whole brain or for segmented tissue (**Fig. 5**). In the case of a whole brain analysis, the peak height and in particular the peak position are governed by (normal-appearing) WM because most pixels are coming from WM, and WM has a higher MTR than gray matter (GM). It is commonly believed that a shift of the peak position reflects global and diffuse changes in WM. Lesions or regional changes of the microstructure would reduce the peak height but not the peak position as long as most regions in WM remain "normal." The peak height can also be affected by cortical atrophy and by partial volume effects because of the very low MTR of cerebrospinal fluid (CSF).

Another approach to measure MTR is region of interest (ROI) analysis, which enables focus on individual MS lesions or on discrete regions in the brain. However, as MS is a diffuse disease, it is virtually impossible to assess the entire brain for disease effects through ROIs. While the regional analysis needs manual interaction and consequently it is biased by the investigator, histogram analysis can be done in a highly automated fashion and therefore it is unbiased. This is particularly important for longitudinal MS studies.

INTERPRETING MAGNETIZATION TRANSFER RATIO CHANGES

Under the assumption that the bound pool is fully saturated, which is however not fully achievable in practice, the MTR becomes a function of the MT rate k_f and the apparent T_1 relaxation time during MT saturation T_{1sat}:[30]

$$MTR = k_f \cdot T_{1sat}$$

Clearly, as a larger macromolecular pool will make the exchange mechanism more efficient, the MTR is expected to strongly depend on the macromolecular density. Nevertheless, the absolute value of the macromolecular pool size can be measured with quantitative MT techniques only.[17–19,31,32]

MS encompasses multiple pathological features including inflammation, edema, demyelination, gliosis, and axonal loss. Only processes that affect the size of the bound proton pool or the water pool are expected to change the MTR, ie, mainly demyelination and edema will have an impact. However, it has been speculated that inflammation per se may also have an effect on the MTR by chancing the physiological environment of the myelin including the accumulation of inflammatory cells.[33] In addition to theoretical considerations there is also convincing support from correlative histopathological studies in MS lesions that indicate the MTR as a strong and independent predictor for the grade of myelination.[34,35] MTR reductions have also been observed in areas of axonal loss; however, as axonal loss occurs mainly in demyelinated areas it is likely that this is mostly a myelin-mediated effect. Otherwise, significant MTR changes have also been observed in the cortex of MS patients, which attests to the wide applicability of this technique for assessing tissue composition.

APPLICATION TO MS
Magnetization Transfer Ratio in Lesions

MT MR imaging has been successfully used to describe the severity of tissue damage in MS lesions both cross-sectionally and longitudinally. It has been observed that MTR drops dramatically when MS lesions start to enhance and that it can show partial or even complete recovery in the subsequent 1 to 6 months.[36–38] As such rapid changes cannot be explained by edema alone, this dynamic is thought to result primarily from de- and remyelination. Hence, MT changes are frequently seen as an ideal means of monitoring this important pathologic process in MS. Evidence for this assumption also comes from the comparison of MTR values with other MR metrics known to reflect the severity of brain tissue damage like the so-called "black holes" on T_1-weighted scans. In this context, MTR was found to be inversely correlated with the degree of T_1 hypointensity and MTR was seen to increase when MS lesions changed from T_1 hypointensity to T_1 isointensity.[38] Histopathologically, this return to T_1 isointensity was shown to correlate with remyelination, whereas persistent T_1 hypointensity was found in demyelinated lesions.[39]

Magnetization Transfer Ratio in Normal-Appearing White Matter

Given the robustness of MTR measurements and the possibility of detecting abnormalities not seen by conventional MR imaging, researchers started to look not only at the changes in MS lesions, but also in WM that appears normal on conventional scans (normal-appearing WM; NAWM). Filippi and colleagues[40] were among the first to note that NAWM close to MS lesions has a reduced MTR. This was especially the case in patients with secondary progressive MS (SPMS). The etiology of this MTR reduction can be manifold. The observation that NAWM MTR abnormalities are more likely and more pronounced with advanced disease suggests secondary phenomena like axonal destruction by Wallerian degeneration and gliosis. On the other hand, there is quite firm evidence that MTR changes precede lesion formation in NAWM. Various researchers have demonstrated MTR reductions in the NAWM as long as 2 years before lesion formation.[41–43] Edema, marked astrocytic proliferation, demyelination, and axonal loss may all account for an increased amount of unbound water in the NAWM and consequently provoke such MTR changes.

MTR analysis of the NAWM has also demonstrated differences in histogram metrics between different phenotypes of MS. Especially patients with primary progressive MS (PPMS) were shown to have a significantly lower histogram peak height with a normal peak position and only a slightly reduced average MTR, which would be in line with the presence of subtle but widespread damage of the NAWM.[44,45] This might in part explain the often observed discrepant finding of advanced disability despite a relatively small number of MS lesions in this disease phenotype in addition to the critical contribution of abnormalities of the spinal cord. Patients with relapsing-remitting MS (RRMS) were consistently shown to have both a lower average MTR and a lower peak height than healthy controls, and these differences were even more pronounced in patients with SPMS.[46,47] These observations indicate the presence of more diffuse damage of the brain WM than one would assume from the observation of disseminated focal MS lesions. In this context, one would especially like to know more about the causality between and the temporal sequence of these events, ie, if such diffuse abnormalities are associated with focal lesions or if they occur independently and if they had preceded MS plaques or if they were their consequence. The reported MTR changes in PPMS, despite the known paucity of WM lesions on conventional MR imaging, strongly argue in favor of an independent phenomenon.

It is still controversial when NAWM MTR abnormalities occur in the evolution of MS. While some researchers found MTR reductions even at the earliest onset of symptomatic MS like in clinically isolated syndromes,[48] other groups could not confirm this finding.[49,50] Although differences in patient selection and in the timing of the examinations cannot be ruled out as possible confounding factors, this could also simply reflect differences in the sensitivity of the imaging techniques used for detecting MT changes.[51] Interestingly, some reduction in normal-appearing brain tissue (NABT)-MTR has been reported even in asymptomatic relatives of patients with MS by some investigators.[52]

Besides these insights into the pathophysiology of MS, the notion of a diffuse damage to the NAWM by MT MR imaging also helps to understand at least part of the so-called "clinico-radiologic paradox," ie, the often striking discrepancy between the amount of visible MS lesions and the level of disability of patients. While various other factors, such as lesion location, lesion severity, and spinal cord damage, are also contributing factors, the role of NAWM cannot be dismissed, especially because it constitutes a large proportion of the brain of MS patients. Diffuse WM changes may be also relevant for MS symptoms that probably originate from a complex disturbance of networks in the brain, like cognitive decline and fatigue.

Magnetization Transfer Ratio in Gray Matter

A reduction of MTR in GM was observed for all clinical phenotypes of MS,[53,54] but more pronounced tissue changes were found especially in patients with SPMS or PPMS.[45] Importantly, only moderate correlations between MTR reductions and WM pathology have been found, which suggests that GM abnormalities are linked only partly to neuronal damage in WM.[55,56] Despite advances in ability to display cortical MS lesions, it is still difficult to know if cortical MTR changes are largely a consequence of yet invisible lesions or rather attest to the presence of diffuse (and possibly coexisting) tissue changes. At any rate, MTR reductions in GM have been found to correlate with cognitive impairment and clinical disability.[56–59] Also, regional MTR values of several cortical areas showed a significant correlation with the Multiple Sclerosis Functional Composite and the Paced Auditory Serial Addition Task scores.[57] However, as no consistent pattern of MTR reductions in various GM structures has been reported, the regional distribution of disease-related tissue changes still remains an open question.[60–62]

Magnetization Transfer Ratio in the Spinal Cord

Spinal cord involvement is a common feature in MS. This is also demonstrated by several studies that showed reduced MTR values in the cervical spinal cord.[63–66] In these studies, the MTR analysis was done using a histogram analysis following semiautomated image segmentation. For several reasons, MT MR imaging in the spinal cord is more challenging than in the brain: the cross-sectional size is small, motion-induced artifacts are more likely, and there is a high probability for partial volume effects from CSF. The low surface area to volume ratio makes segmentation quite critical in particular in the presence of atrophy. All these factors may bias histogram analysis and should be considered when comparing MTR results from different studies.

Magnetization Transfer MR Imaging in Treatment Trials of Multiple Sclerosis

Because of its relative ease of application and its high sensitivity, MT MR imaging is increasingly used in the evaluation and follow-up of MS patients including treatment trials. In the European Study of Intravenous Immunoglobulin (IVIG) in SPMS, no MTR change over 2 years was observed following treatment, while the placebo-treated patients showed a significant drop of the MTR peak height of normal-appearing brain tissue.[67] It was speculated that this might support a disease-stabilizing effect of IVIG. From the comparison with MTR measurements in another trial of SPMS,[68] it also becomes clear that it is important to use a standardized MT protocol across different centers and, in addition, to correct statistically for system-related MTR effects. In this context, it has been shown recently that B_1, which is the strength of the RF field used for saturation, plays a dominant role.[69] This can be explained by the fact that the MTR is directly related to the power of the saturation pulse. Therefore, any deviation from the nominal value of the RF saturation pulse, owing to inhomogeneities of the active B_1 field or owing to different coil concepts, impacts significantly on the results and contributes to intercenter variability irrespective of identical imaging protocols. With the help of B_1 maps it is possible to correct for these scanner-related center effects.[69] Attempts to create a robust phantom for the standardization of the MTR across centers have unfortunately remained unsuccessful so far.

SUMMARY

Because of its sensitivity for microstructural tissue changes, MT MR imaging has provided significant insights into the focal and diffuse CNS abnormalities associated with MS. MT MR imaging has especially revealed tissue changes that have not been recognized by conventional MR sequences before. Although MS is usually conceived as a multifocal disease, MT MR imaging has also largely contributed to the recognition of a further disease process, which is rather diffuse. This has sparked new concepts and theories although it is not yet clear how this finding can be incorporated into our pathophysiologic understanding of the disease. Otherwise, MT MR imaging does not yet appear to be able to contribute to individual patient management and has not gained a role in clinical practice. Thus far, the use of MT MR imaging in clinical trials has also been disappointing. However, this may be related to the inefficacy of the drugs tested and the initial technical difficulties observed with multicenter trials rather than to the potential of MT MR imaging. Possibilities and recommendations for the standardization of MT MR imaging are thus of paramount importance. Further progress may also be expected from strategies that allow assessment of MT in a more quantitative manner such as by mapping other fundamental MT parameters of the two-pool model. Such more detailed insights might not only add to our pathophysiologic knowledge, but could contribute further to determining and better understanding of the treatment effects of available and newly developed drugs for MS.

REFERENCES

1. Wolff SD, Balaban RS. Magnetization transfer contrast (MTC) and tissue water proton relaxation in vivo. Magn Reson Med 1989;10:135–44.
2. Eng J, Ceckler TL, Balaban RS. Quantitative 1H magnetization transfer imaging in vivo. Magn Reson Med 1991;17:304–14.
3. Wolff SD, Balaban RS. Magnetization transfer imaging: practical aspects and clinical applications. Radiology 1994;192:593–9.
4. Morrison C, Henkelman RM. A model for magnetization transfer in tissues. Magn Reson Med 1995;33:475–82.
5. Harrison R, Bronskill J, Henkelman RM. Magnetization transfer and T2 relaxation components. Magn Reson Med 1995;33:490–6.
6. Lancaster JL, Andrews T, Hardies LJ, et al. Three-pool model of white matter. J Magn Reson Imaging 2003;17:1–10.
7. Portnoy S, Stanisz G. Is a two-pool MT model valid in tissues with multicomponent T2? Proc.of the International Society for Magnetic Resonance in Medicine, 14th scientific meeting, Seattle, 1996. p. 2110.
8. Stanisz GJ, Kecojevic A, Bronskill MJ, et al. Characterizing white matter with magnetization transfer and T2. Magn Reson Med 1999;42:1128–36.
9. Vavasour IM, Whittall KP, Li DK, et al. Different magnetization transfer effects exhibited by the short and long T2 components in human brain. Magn Reson Med 2000;44:860–6.
10. Otting G, Liepinsh E, Wüthrich K. Protein hydration in aqueous solution. Science 1991;254:974–80.
11. Liepinsh E, Otting G, Wütrich K. NMR spectroscopy of hydroxyl protons in aqueous solutions of peptides and proteins. J Biomol NMR 1992;2:447–65.
12. Denisov VP, Halle B. Hydrogen exchange and protein hydration: the deuteron spin relaxation dispersions of BPTI and ubiquitin. J Mol Biol 1995;245:698–709.
13. Kakalis LT, Baianu IC. Oxygen-17 and deuterium nuclear magnetic relaxation studies of lysozyme hydration in solution: field dispersion, concentration, pH/pD, and protein activity dependencies. Arch Biochem Biopys 1988;287:829–41.
14. Ceckler TL, Balaban RS. Tritium-proton magnetization transfer as a probe of cross-relaxation in aqueous lipid bilayer suspension. J Magn Reson 1991;93:572–88.
15. Hills BP, Favret FA. A comparative multinuclear relaxation study of protein-DSMO and protein water-water interaction. J Magn Reson B 1994;103:142–51.
16. Kucharczyk W, MacDonald PM, Stanisz GJ, et al. Relaxivity and magnetization transfer of white matter lipids at MR imaging: importance of cerebrosides and pH. Radiology 1994;192:521–9.
17. Sled JG, Pike GB. Quantitative imaging of magnetization transfer exchange and relaxation properties in vivo using MRI. Magn Reson Med 2001;46:923–31.
18. Ramani A, Dalton C, Miller DH, et al. Precise estimate of fundamental in-vivo MT parameters in human brain in clinically feasible times. Magn Reson Imaging 2002;20:721–31.
19. Yarnykh VL. Pulsed Z-spectroscopic imaging of cross-relaxation parameters in tissues for human MRI: theory and clinical applications. Magn Reson Med 2002;47:929–39.
20. Hua J, Hurst GC. Analysis of on- and off-resonance magnetization transfer techniques. J Magn Reson Imaging 1995;5:113–9.
21. Pachot-Clouard M, Darrasse L. Optimization of T2-selective binomial pulses for magnetization transfer. Magn Reson Med 1995;34:462–9.
22. Schick F. Pulsed magnetization transfer contrast MRI by a sequence with water selective excitation. J Comput Assist Tomogr 1996;20:73–9.
23. Barker GJ, Tofts PS, Gass A. An interleaved sequence for accurate and reproducible clinical measurement of magnetization transfer ratio. Magn Reson Imag 1996;14:403–11.
24. Bieri O, Scheffler K. On magnetization transfer and balanced SSFP. Proc.of the International Society for Magnetic Resonance in Medicine, 15th scientific meeting, Berlin, 2007.
25. Finelli DA, Hurst GC, Amantia P, et al. Cerebral white matter: technical development and clinical applications of effective magnetization transfer (MT) power

concepts for high-power, thin-section, quantitative MT examinations. Radiology 1996;199:219–26.

26. Fazekas F, Ropele S, Enzinger C, et al. MTI of white matter hyperintensities. Brain 2005;128:2926–32.

27. Ropele S, Enzinger C, Reishofer G, et al. Fast three-dimensional magnetization transfer imaging at 3T. Proc.of the International Society for Magnetic Resonance in Medicine, 15th scientific meeting, Berlin, 2007.

28. van Buchem MA, Udupa JK, McGowan JC, et al. Global volumetric estimation of disease burden in multiple sclerosis based on magnetization transfer imaging. AJNR Am J Neuroradiol 1997;18:1287–90.

29. van Buchem MA, McGowan JC, Kolson DL, et al. Quantitative volumetric magnetization transfer analysis in multiple sclerosis: estimation of macroscopic and microscopic disease burden. Magn Reson Med 1996;36:632–6.

30. Forsen S, Hoffman A. A study of moderately rapid chemical exchange reactions by means of nuclear magnetic double resonance. J Chem Phys 1963; 39:2892–901.

31. Gochberg DF, Kennan RP, Robson MD, et al. Quantitative imaging of magnetization transfer using multiple selective pulses. Magn Reson Med 1999;41:1065–72.

32. Ropele S, Seifert T, Enzinger C, et al. Method for quantitative imaging of the macromolecular 1H fraction in tissues. Magn Reson Med 2003;49: 864–71.

33. Gareau PJ, Rutt BK, Karlik SJ, et al. Magnetization transfer and multicomponent T2 relaxation measurements with histopathologic correlation in an experimental model of MS. J Magn Reson Imaging 2000; 11:586–95.

34. Schmierer K, Scaravilli F, Altmann DR, et al. Magnetization transfer ratio and myelin in postmortem multiple sclerosis brain. Ann Neurol 2004;56:407–15.

35. Schmierer K, Wheeler-Kingshott CA, Tozer DJ, et al. Quantitative magnetic resonance of postmortem multiple sclerosis brain before and after fixation. Magn Reson Med 2008;59:268–77.

36. Dousset V, Gayou A, Brochet B, et al. Early structural changes in acute MS lesions assessed by serial magnetization transfer studies. Neurology 1998;51: 1150–5.

37. Filippi M, Rocca M, Comi G. Magnetization transfer ratios of multiple sclerosis lesions with variable durations of enhancement. J Neurol Sci 1998;159:162–5.

38. van Waesberghe JH, van Walderveen MA, Castelijns JA, et al. Patterns of lesion development in multiple sclerosis: longitudinal observations with T1-weighted spin-echo and magnetization transfer MR. AJNR Am J Neuroradiol 1998;19:675–83.

39. Bitsch A, Kuhlmann T, Stadelmann C, et al. A longitudinal MRI study of histopathologically defined hypointense multiple sclerosis lesions. Ann Neurol 2001;49:793–6.

40. Filippi M, et al. A magnetisation transfer imaging study of normal-appearing white matter in multiple sclerosis. Neurology 1995;45:478–82.

41. Pike GB, De Stefano N, Narayanan S, et al. Magnetization transfer MR imaging of white matter before lesion appearance on T2-weighted images. Radiology 2000;215:824–30.

42. Filippi M, Rocca MA, Martino G, et al. Magnetization transfer changes in the normal appearing white matter precede the appearance of enhancing lesions in patients with multiple sclerosis. Ann Neurol 1998;43: 809–14.

43. Goodkin DE, Rooney WD, Sloan R, et al. A serial study of new MS lesions and the white matter from which they arise. Neurology 1998;51:1689–97.

44. Filippi M, Iannucci G, Tortorella C, et al. Comparison of MS clinical phenotypes using conventional and magnetization transfer MRI. Neurology 1999;52: 588–94.

45. Rovaris M, Bozzali M, Santuccio G, et al. In vivo assessment of the brain and cervical cord pathology of patients with primary progressive multiple sclerosis. Brain 2001;124:2540–9.

46. Filippi M, Inglese M, Rovaris M, et al. Magnetization transfer imaging to monitor the evolution of MS: a 1-year follow-up study. Neurology 2000;55:940–6.

47. Kalkers NF, Hintzen RQ, van Waesberghe JH, et al. Magnetization transfer histogram parameters reflect all dimensions of MS pathology, including atrophy. J Neurol Sci 2001;184:155–62.

48. Iannucci G, Tortorella C, Rovaris M, et al. Prognostic value of MR and magnetization transfer imaging findings in patients with clinically isolated syndromes suggestive of multiple sclerosis at presentation. AJNR Am J Neuroradiol 2000;21:1034–8.

49. Kaiser JS, Grossman RI, Polansky M, et al. Magnetization transfer histogram analysis of monosymptomatic episodes of neurologic dysfunction: preliminary findings. AJNR Am J Neuroradiol 2000;21:1043–7.

50. Brex PA, Leary SM, Plant GT, et al. Magnetization transfer imaging in patients with clinically isolated syndromes suggestive of multiple sclerosis. AJNR Am J Neuroradiol 2001;22:947–51.

51. Traboulsee A, Dehmeshki J, Brex PA, et al. Normal-appearing brain tissue MTR histograms in clinically isolated syndromes suggestive of MS. Neurology 2002;59:126–8.

52. Siger-Zajdel M, Filippi M, Selmaj K. MTR discloses subtle changes in the normal-appearing tissue from relatives of patients with MS. Neurology 2002; 58:317–20.

53. Fernando KT, Tozer DJ, Miszkiel KA, et al. Magnetization transfer histograms in clinically isolated syndromes suggestive of multiple sclerosis. Brain 2005;128:2911–25.

54. Davies GR, Altmann DR, Hadjiprocopis A, et al. Increasing normal-appearing grey and white matter

magnetisation transfer ratio abnormality in early relapsing-remitting multiple sclerosis. J Neurol 2005; 252:1037–44.

55. Cercignani M, Bozzali M, Iannucci G, et al. Magnetisation transfer ratio and mean diffusivity of normal-appearing white and gray matter from patients with multiple sclerosis. J Neurol Neurosurg Psychiatr 2001;70:311–7.

56. Ge Y, Grossman RI, Udupa JK, et al. Magnetization transfer ratio histogram analysis of gray matter in relapsing-remitting multiple sclerosis. AJNR Am J Neuroradiol 2001;22:470–5.

57. Ranjeva JP, Audoin B, Au Duong MV, et al. Local tissue damage assessed with statistical mapping analysis of brain magnetization transfer ratio: relationship with functional status of patients in the earliest stage of multiple sclerosis. AJNR Am J Neuroradiol 2005;26:119–27.

58. Rovaris M, Filippi M, Minicucci L, et al. Cortical/subcortical disease burden and cognitive impairment in patients with multiple sclerosis. AJNR Am J Neuroradiol 2000;21:402–8.

59. Dehmeshki J, Chard DT, Leary SM, et al. The normal appearing gray matter in primary progressive multiple sclerosis: a magnetisation transfer imaging study. J Neurol 2003;250:67–74.

60. Davies GR, Altmann DR, Rashid W, et al. Emergence of thalamic magnetization transfer ratio abnormality in early relapsing-remitting multiple sclerosis. Mult Scler 2005;11:276–81.

61. Audoin B, Ranjeva JP, Au Duong MV, et al. Voxel-based analysis of MTR images: a method to locate grey matter abnormalities in patients at the earliest stage of multiple sclerosis. J Magn Reson Imaging 2005;20:765–71.

62. Sharma J, Zivadinov R, Jaisani Z, et al. A magnetization transfer MRI study of deep gray matter involvement in multiple sclerosis. J Neuroimaging 2006;16:302–10.

63. Bozzali M, Rocca MA, Iannucci G, et al. Magnetization-transfer histogram analysis of the cervical cord in patients with multiple sclerosis. AJNR Am J Neuroradiol 1999;20:1803–8.

64. Lycklama à Nijeholt GJ, Castelijns JA, Lazeron RH, et al. Magnetization transfer ratio of the spinal cord in multiple sclerosis: relationship to atrophy and neurologic disability. J Neuroimaging 2000;10:67–72.

65. Filippi M, Bozzali M, Horsfield MA, et al. A conventional and magnetization transfer MRI study of the cervical cord in patients with MS. Neurology 2000; 54:207–13.

66. Rovaris M, Gallo A, Riva R, et al. An MT MRI study of the cervical cord in clinically isolated syndromes suggestive of MS. Neurology 2004;63:584–5.

67. Filippi M, Rocca MA, Pagani E, et al. European study on intravenous immunoglobulin in multiple sclerosis: results of magnetization transfer magnetic resonance imaging analysis. Arch Neurol 2004;61: 1409–12.

68. Inglese M, van Waesberghe JH, Rovaris M, et al. The effect of interferon beta-1b on quantities derived from MT MRI in secondary progressive MS. Neurology 2003;60:853–60.

69. Ropele S, Filippi M, Valsasina P, et al. Assessment and correction of B1-induced errors in magnetization transfer ratio measurements. Magn Reson Med 2005;53:134–40.

Diffusion Tensor MR Imaging

Marco Rovaris, MD[a,b], Federica Agosta, MD[a],
Elisabetta Pagani, PhD[a], Massimo Filippi, MD[a],*

KEYWORDS

- Multiple selerosis • Diffusion tensor MR imaging
- Normal-appearing white matter
- Gray matter • Tractography

Diffusion MR imaging has been largely used to study multiple sclerosis (MS), because of its ability to detect and quantify disease-related pathology of the central nervous system (CNS).[1] The characteristics of diffusion, which can be defined as the random translational motion of molecules in a fluid system, are influenced by several CNS tissue components, including cell membranes and organelles.[2] The MR imaging–measured diffusion coefficient of healthy CNS tissues is, therefore, lower than that in free water; it is called the apparent diffusion coefficient (ADC).[2] Pathologic processes that result in a decrease of restricting barriers can determine an increase of the ADC values.[2] Because the magnitude of diffusion also depends on the direction in which it is measured, its full characterization can be obtained in terms of a diffusion tensor (DT),[3] a matrix that accounts for the correlation existing between molecular displacement along orthogonal directions. From the DT, it is possible to derive some parameters, which are quantitative and invariant to the frame choice: the mean diffusivity (MD), which measures the average molecular motion independent of any tissue directionality, and some other dimensionless indices of anisotropic diffusion, including fractional anisotropy (FA), which reflect the prevalence of diffusivity along one spatial direction (eg, along axonal fibers rather than perpendicular to them).[3] The main postmortem correlates of diffusivity changes in MS are demyelination and axonal loss.[4,5] Correlation with pathologic features is stronger for anisotropy than for diffusivity indices in the brain[5] and spinal cord[4] of patients who have MS.

This article discusses the main clinical applications of DT MR imaging to the study of MS and the role of new acquisition schemes and postprocessing methods.

DIFFUSION TENSOR MR IMAGING FEATURES OF MULTIPLE SCLEROSIS–RELATED TISSUE DAMAGE

In MS, the first diffusion MR imaging studies[6] consistently reported increased ADC values within both T2-visible lesions and the normal-appearing white matter (NAWM). These studies were affected by several limitations, however, including limited brain coverage, low number of encoded directions, and high susceptibility to motion artifacts. During the subsequent years, thanks to the development of more sophisticated acquisition schemes and the application of novel postprocessing techniques, DT MR imaging has been increasingly applied to the study of MS-related tissue damage with encouraging results.

DT MR imaging has proved to be a valuable tool for investigating the variety of pathologic features of T2-visible lesions. In focal lesions, diffusion abnormalities (ie, increased MD and decreased FA) are always more pronounced than in the NAWM; however, their values are highly heterogeneous (see Ref[1] for a review). The more severe abnormalities have been found in T1 hypointense lesions (also known as "black holes"),[7–9] which represent areas of irreversible tissue disruption, gliosis, and axonal loss. Conversely, when comparing enhancing versus nonenhancing lesions,[7–10] conflicting results have been reported; hence, how much DT

[a] Neuroimaging Research Unit, Department of Neurology, San Raffaele Scientific Institute and University, Via Olgettina, 60-20132, Milan, Italy
[b] Multiple Sclerosis Unit, Scientific Institute Santa Maria Nascente—Fondazione Don Gnocchi, Milan, Italy
* Corresponding author.
E-mail address: filippi.massimo@hsr.it (M. Filippi).

Neuroimag Clin N Am 19 (2009) 37–43
doi:10.1016/j.nic.2008.08.001
1052-5149/08/$ – see front matter © 2008 Elsevier Inc. All rights reserved.

MR imaging–detectable tissue disorganization within acute lesions is permanent (ie, related to neurodegeneration) and how much is transient (ie, related to edema, demyelination, and remyelination) remains an unsolved issue. A longitudinal study of enhancing MS lesions, which were followed up for 1 to 3 months,[10] has shown that MD values were increased in all lesions, but continued to increase during follow-up only in a subgroup of them. This finding highlights that contrast enhancement does not allow us to profile acute MS lesions that are characterized by varying degrees of tissue disruption. In the same study,[10] increased MD values were correlated with a greater degree of T1 hypointensity. Interestingly, a recent DT MR imaging study[11] showed that cortical lesions have higher FA values than the normal-appearing gray matter (GM). This paradoxical finding may actually reflect the intralesional loss of dendrites and activation of microglial cells, thereby highlighting the potential contribution of DT MR imaging to help disentangle the pathologic features of GM lesions.[11] More recently,[12] the relationship between T2 relaxation times and DT MR imaging measures was investigated in a sample of MS lesions: lesions with long T2 fraction demonstrated the most pronounced diffusivity abnormalities, which were highly correlated with decreased myelin water content. When considered together, these findings support the notion that DT MR imaging may represent a technique able to assess the severity of functionally relevant tissue damage within MS lesions.

Outside T2 lesions, DT MR imaging discloses the presence of abnormalities in the NAWM and GM of patients who have MS,[1] even before the development of new plaques.[13] DT MR imaging is likely to be sensitive to the more disabling features of MS pathology in the NAWM, because diffusion abnormalities are more pronounced with increasing disease duration and neurologic impairment.[14–17] NAWM and GM damage is only partially correlated with the extent of focal lesions and the severity of intrinsic lesion damage,[1] suggesting that diffusivity changes in normal-appearing tissues are not entirely dependent on retrograde degeneration of axons transected in T2-visible lesions. The results of a recent study[18] correlating diffusivity measures with perfusion findings in the corpus callosum of patients who had relapsing-remitting (RR) MS are more consistent with what would be seen in primary ischemia than in secondary hypoperfusion attributable to Wallerian degeneration.

DT MR imaging is also useful to assess the evolution of MS damage over time.[16,19,20] Changes of DT MR imaging metrics seem to be independent of the concomitant accumulation of T2 lesions and reduction of brain tissue volume.[16,19,20] Moreover, DT MR

imaging might be more sensitive to detect the accrual of GM damage than that of NAWM,[16,19] because it is the earliest clinical stage of MS.[21] The application of DT MR imaging in monitoring the evolution of MS-related tissue damage over time therefore holds promise for trials aiming at assessing the efficacy of neuroprotective therapies.

CLINICAL CORRELATIONS

DT MR imaging features and clinical severity of patients who have established MS are shown to be interrelated, the strongest associations being those related to the diffusion characteristics of T2 lesions[13] and GM.[14,22–24] The absence or mildness of DT MR imaging abnormalities in the normal-appearing brain may accompany a favorable clinical status, as suggested in patients who have pediatric MS.[25] Because the accumulation of damage in focal lesions and NAWM occurs even during the earliest nondisabling phases of MS[17,26] and this does not seem to be the case, at least at the same extent, for GM, GM diffusivity changes may be viewed as a hallmark of the more disabling and progressive stages of the disease.[21,22] GM diffusivity features have also been related to the neuropsychologic profile of patients who have MS.[22,24] In patients who had the benign form of MS, the severity of GM damage associated with cognitive impairment was similar to that observed in patients who had progressive MS and irreversible locomotor disability.[24] Two other studies[27,28] correlated DT MR imaging findings with the presence and severity of fatigue in patients who had MS. Disappointingly, the average MD and FA from brain, GM, and T2 lesions were not different between fatigued and nonfatigued patients, nor there was a correlation between any of these quantities and the fatigue severity scale scores.[27,28] Apart from being used as stand-alone paraclinical measures, DT MR imaging can contribute to composite MR-based scores able to explain a large part of the variance of MS-related disability.[17,29] Moreover, the results of a follow-up study of patients who had primary progressive (PP) MS[30] suggest that the severity of diffusion abnormalities in GM may predict disability worsening 5 years later. Further larger, prospective studies are now warranted to ascertain whether DT MR imaging–derived measures of tissue damage might be used as paraclinical markers of MS prognosis.

NOVEL STRATEGIES
Diffusion Tensor MR Imaging of the Optic Nerves and Spinal Cord

Diffusion imaging of the optic nerve and spinal cord are technically more challenging than that of the brain, and studies of these structures are therefore still limited.[1] The development of novel DT MR imaging sequences has recently made it possible to achieve an accurate estimate of the extent of damage in these regions, however.[20,31–38] In the optic nerve, DT MR imaging measures provide an indication of the structural integrity of axons, and are correlated with neurophysiologic findings and, at a lesser magnitude, with clinical measures of visual functioning.[31,32] DT MR imaging of the cervical cord provides measures of the global diffusivity and anisotropy status in this structure, which is known to play a major role for the locomotor abilities of patients who have MS. A DT MR imaging study of the cervical cord of patients who had RRMS and secondary progressive (SP) MS has shown that patients who have MS have MD and FA histogram characteristics suggestive of diffuse cord damage.[33] In the same study,[33] a multivariate linear regression model retained cord average FA and brain average MD as variables independently influencing patients' clinical disability. Patients who have PPMS also have abnormal diffusivity and anisotropy of the cervical cord.[34] When compared with SPMS,[36] patients who had benign MS showed a milder cervical cord damage. Moreover, in patients who had benign MS, both cord cross-sectional area and FA were factors independently associated with the degree of clinical disability,[36] thus suggesting that DT MR imaging may contribute to a comprehensive assessment of spinal cord damage. Likewise, DT MR imaging of the cervical cord may contribute to better characterized spinal cord damage of Devic neuromyelitis optica.[37] Recently, a 2-year follow-up conventional and DT MR imaging study involving a large cohort of patients who had MS[20] showed that both progressive atrophy and damage to the remaining tissue occur in the cervical cord. These two components of cord damage were not strictly interrelated. MS cord pathology was also found to be independent of concomitant brain changes, to develop at different rates according to disease phenotype, and to be associated with medium-term disability accrual.[20] Cervical cord DT MR imaging in combination with proton MR spectroscopy has also been found to provide a reliable account of the cord damage occurring in patients who have spinal relapses.[38]

Tractography

DT MR imaging tractography exploits the fact that axonal structures constitute a barrier to water diffusion, making it much more free along the axis of the fibers than perpendicular to it.[39] By tracking the principal diffusion direction (ie, the direction of the primary eigenvector of the DT), nervous pathways can be reconstructed.[39] DT MR imaging tractography, therefore, is a promising technique for in vivo segmentation of the major WM tracts in the brain (**Fig. 1**).[39] Some limitations prevent tractography algorithms from reconstructing the correct trajectories when more complex architectures than a single orientationally coherent fiber bundle are assessed. One of these limitations is intrinsic to the use of the tensor to model the diffusion process, which causes the principal diffusion direction not to follow the "real" fiber axes when fibers cross, but rather a direction that is the result of averaging between these crossing fibers.[40] The poor spatial resolution of echo planar imaging, at present the most widely used technique for DT MR imaging, and the low signal-to-noise ratio of the acquired data also contribute to making the correct reconstruction of fiber bundles a challenging task.[40] Furthermore, the application of tractography to the study of patients who have MS suffers from the drawback that the disease causes both focal and diffuse alterations of tissue organization, which result in a decreased anisotropy and a consequent increase in uncertainty of the primary eigenvector of the DT.[40] A possible approach to overcome this problem is the use of probability maps of tracts of interest obtained from healthy subjects

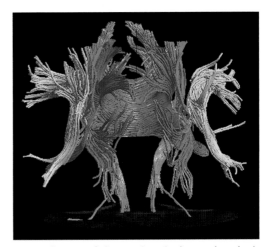

Fig. 1. Behavior of the corticospinal tract (cyan), the corpus callosum (magenta), and the superior longitudinal fasciculus (yellow) as reconstructed by a streamline tractography algorithm in a healthy subject. (*From* Pagani E, Filippi M, Rocca MA, et al. A method for obtaining tract-specific diffusion tensor MRI measurements in the presence of disease: application to patients with clinically isolated syndromes suggestive of multiple sclerosis. Neuroimage 2005;26:258–65; with permission.)

to assess DT MR imaging metrics from the corresponding patients' tracts.[41]

In patients who have MS, diffusivity and anisotropy of the corticospinal tracts (CST) correlate with clinical measures of locomotor disability, such as the expanded disability status scale score or the pyramidal functional system score at this scale, more than T2 lesion burden and the overall extent of diffusivity changes of the brain.[42,43] The analysis of DT eigenvalues of the CST of patients who have RRMS has suggested Wallerian degeneration as the main mechanisms underlying diffusion changes in this WM structure.[44] Moreover, a DT MR imaging tractography study of patients who had clinically isolated syndromes suggestive of MS showed that those patients who had motor impairment had increased MD and T2 lesion volume in the CST compared with those patients who did not have pyramidal symptoms.[41] In patients who have MS, ADC values of the corpus callosum are associated with the level of cognitive performance.[43] A DT MR imaging tractography study of patients who had optic neuritis showed reduced connectivity values in both left and right optic radiations compared with controls, suggesting the occurrence of transsynaptic degeneration secondary to optic nerve damage.[45] DT MR imaging tractography also provided a method to identify NAWM fibers at risk for degeneration because they intersect focal T2-visible lesions.[46]

Tract-specific abnormalities of the CST were investigated using a multiparametric approach, which included diffusion-based tractography, magnetization transfer (MT) MR imaging, and T2 relaxation times in a large cohort of patients who had MS.[47] On average, tract profiles were different between patients and controls, particularly in the subcortical WM and corona radiata, for all indices examined except for FA.[47] In patients who had RRMS, CST tissue damage measured using DT MR imaging tractography was associated with altered movement-associated functional effective connectivity.[48] Similarly, patients who had benign MS showed a correlation between diffusivity changes of the corpus callosum and abnormal interhemispheric effective connectivity during the performance of attention-related tasks.[49]

Voxelwise Analysis

Voxelwise approaches to the analysis of quantitative MR imaging data, such as voxel-based morphometry,[50] hold promise to improve our ability to study the structural features of MS damage, because they assess the presence and quantify the extent of brain damage topographically. Voxel-based MR imaging studies of patients

who have MS have been so far mainly focused on measures of atrophy,[51] but this approach may represent a valid option also for the analysis of DT MR imaging data. For instance, using a voxel-based approach, a recent study[52] showed that patients who have RR and benign MS differ in topographic distribution of WM damage, whereas no between-group differences were found when the overall extent of WM diffusivity changes was assessed (**Fig. 2**). These findings support the notion that the assessment of regional damage using DT MR imaging may be more rewarding than that of "global" brain damage to gain insight into the relation between clinical status and disease burden in MS. More recently, a voxel-based method to obtain estimates of WM fiber bundle volumes using DT MR imaging was developed;[53] the method estimates an index of volume changes derived from the transformation between an FA atlas based on the morphologic characteristics of a reference population and an individual subject FA map. This approach has been successfully applied to the assessment of the topographic distribution of age-related WM volume changes in healthy subjects,[54] and might be helpful to better depict the pathologic changes associated with MS.

UNRESOLVED ISSUES AND FUTURE PERSPECTIVES

Too little is still known about the actual features underlying diffusion changes in MS. On the other hand, some pieces of evidence suggest that the various, and often concomitant, pathologic abnormalities occurring in the MS brain might affect the diffusivity and anisotropy characteristics of tissues in opposite ways, thereby complicating the interpretation of DT MR imaging findings.[55] These aspects have to be carefully considered before interrogating DT MR imaging in the differential diagnosis between MS and other demyelinating disorders.[37,56,57]

The best acquisition and postprocessing strategies for MS studies also remain a matter of debate.[40] The inter-scanner variability of DT MR imaging measures and the issues related to high field scanner acquisitions (such as those associated with our increased chemical shift and with susceptibility artifacts) warrant further investigation. Moreover, some limitations of DT tractography, which may lead to erroneous fiber tracing, still need to be overcome by technical development. The contribution of newer and more sophisticated techniques to DT MR imaging investigations of MS also needs to be evaluated.[40] Among these techniques, high *b*-value q-space imaging[58] holds promise to increase the sensitivity of

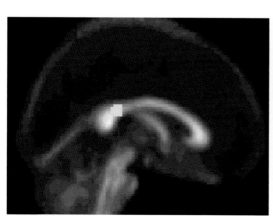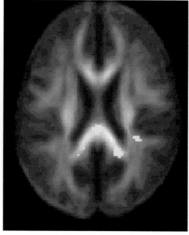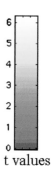

t values

Fig. 2. Voxelwise analysis of fractional anisotropy (FA) maps in patients who have benign MS. Clusters of significantly decreased FA in the splenium of the corpus callosum and temporal fibers in patients who have benign MS compared with control subjects are mapped over the FA template. (*From* Ceccarelli A, Rocca MA, Pagani E, et al. The topographical distribution of tissue injury in benign MS: a 3T multiparametric study. Neuroimage 2008;39:1499–509; with permission.)

"conventional," low *b*-value DT MR imaging in the detection of NAWM abnormalities.

The precision and accuracy of DT MR imaging scans in detecting longitudinal, MS-related changes also need to be defined and ad hoc large-scale, prospective studies are warranted. This issue is central for a future application of DT MR imaging to the monitoring of the disease evolution in MS clinical trials and, eventually, in the assessment of individual patients.

REFERENCES

1. Rovaris M, Gass A, Bammer R, et al. Diffusion MRI in multiple sclerosis. Neurology 2005;65:1526–32.
2. Le Bihan D, Breton E, Lallemand D, et al. MR imaging of intravoxel incoherent motions: application to diffusion and perfusion in neurologic disorders. Radiology 1986;161:401–7.
3. Pierpaoli C, Jezzard P, Basser PJ, et al. Diffusion tensor MR imaging of the human brain. Radiology 1996;201:637–48.
4. Mottershead JP, Schmierer K, Clemence M, et al. High field MRI correlates of myelin content and axonal density in multiple sclerosis—a post-mortem study of the spinal cord. J Neurol 2003;250:1293–301.
5. Schmierer K, Wheeler-Kingshott CA, Boulby PA, et al. Diffusion tensor imaging of *post mortem* multiple sclerosis brain. Neuroimage 2007;35:467–77.
6. Horsfield MA, Larsson HB, Jones DK, et al. Diffusion magnetic resonance imaging in multiple sclerosis. J Neurol Neurosurg Psychiatr 1998;64(Suppl 1):S80–4.
7. Filippi M, Iannucci G, Cercignani M, et al. A quantitative study of water diffusion in multiple sclerosis lesions and normal-appearing white matter using echo-planar imaging. Arch Neurol 2000;57:1017–21.
8. Filippi M, Cercignani M, Inglese M, et al. Diffusion tensor magnetic resonance imaging in multiple sclerosis. Neurology 2001;56:304–11.
9. Bammer R, Augustin M, Strasser-Fuchs S, et al. Magnetic resonance diffusion tensor imaging for characterizing diffuse and focal white matter abnormalities in multiple sclerosis. Magn Reson Med 2000;44:583–9.
10. Castriota Scanderbeg A, Sabatini U, Fasano F, et al. Diffusion of water in large demyelinating lesions: a follow-up study. Neuroradiology 2002;44:764–7.
11. Poonawalla AH, Hasan KM, Gupta RK, et al. Diffusion-tensor MR imaging of cortical lesions in multiple sclerosis: initial findings. Radiology 2008;246:880–6.
12. Kolind SH, Laule C, Vavasour IM, et al. Complementary information from multi-exponential T2 relaxation and diffusion tensor imaging reveals differences between multiple sclerosis lesions. Neuroimage 2008;40:77–85.
13. Rocca MA, Cercignani M, Iannucci G, et al. Weekly diffusion-weighted imaging of normal-appearing white matter in MS. Neurology 2000;55:882–4.
14. Bozzali M, Cercignani M, Sormani MP, et al. Quantification of brain gray matter damage in different MS phenotypes by use of diffusion tensor MR imaging. AJNR Am J Neuroradiol 2002;23:985–8.
15. Rovaris M, Bozzali M, Iannucci G, et al. Assessment of normal-appearing white and grey matter in patients with primary progressive multiple sclerosis. Arch Neurol 2002;59:1406–12.

16. Rovaris M, Gallo A, Valsasina P, et al. Short-term accrual of gray matter pathology in patients with progressive multiple sclerosis: an in vivo study using diffusion tensor MRI. Neuroimage 2005;24:1139–46.

17. Pulizzi A, Rovaris M, Judica E, et al. Determinants of disability in multiple sclerosis at various disease stages: a multiparametric magnetic resonance study. Arch Neurol 2007;64:1163–8.

18. Saindane AM, Law M, Ge Y, et al. Correlation of diffusion tensor and dynamic perfusion MR imaging metrics in normal-appearing corpus callosum: support for primary hypoperfusion in multiple sclerosis. AJNR Am J Neuroradiol 2007;28:767–72.

19. Oreja-Guevara C, Rovaris M, Iannucci G, et al. Progressive grey matter damage in patients with relapsing-remitting MS: a longitudinal diffusion tensor MRI study. Arch Neurol 2005;62:578–84.

20. Agosta F, Absinta M, Sormani MP, et al. In vivo assessment of cervical cord damage in MS patients: a longitudinal diffusion tensor MRI study. Brain 2007; 130:2111–9.

21. Rovaris M, Judica E, Ceccarelli A, et al. A 3-year diffusion tensor MRI study of grey matter damage progression during the earliest clinical stage of MS. J Neurol 2008, in press.

22. Rovaris M, Iannucci G, Falautano M, et al. Cognitive dysfunction in patients with mildly disabling relapsing-remitting multiple sclerosis: an exploratory study with diffusion tensor MR imaging. J Neurol Sci 2002; 195:103–9.

23. Vrenken H, Pouwels PJ, Geurts JJ, et al. Altered diffusion tensor in multiple sclerosis normal-appearing brain tissue: cortical diffusion changes seem related to clinical deterioration. J Magn Reson Imaging 2006;23:628–36.

24. Rovaris M, Riccitelli G, Judica E, et al. Cognitive impairment and structural brain damage in benign multiple sclerosis. Neurology, in press.

25. Tortorella C, Rocca MA, Mezzapesa D, et al. MRI quantification of gray and white matter damage in patients with early-onset multiple sclerosis. J Neurol 2006;253:903–7.

26. Gallo A, Rovaris M, Riva R, et al. Diffusion tensor MRI detects normal-appearing white matter damage unrelated to short-term disease activity in patients at the earlier stage of multiple sclerosis. Arch Neurol 2005;62:803–8.

27. Codella M, Rocca MA, Colombo B, et al. Cerebral grey matter pathology and fatigue in patients with multiple sclerosis: a preliminary study. J Neurol Sci 2002;194:71–4.

28. Codella M, Rocca MA, Colombo B, et al. A preliminary study of magnetization transfer and diffusion tensor MRI of multiple sclerosis patients with fatigue. J Neurol 2002;249:535–7.

29. Mainero C, De Stefano N, Iannucci G, et al. Correlates of MS disability assessed in vivo using aggregates of MR quantities. Neurology 2001;56: 1331–4.

30. Rovaris M, Judica E, Gallo A, et al. Grey matter damage predicts the evolution of primary progressive multiple sclerosis at 5 years. Brain 2006;129: 2628–34.

31. Hickman SJ, Wheeler-Kingshott CA, Jones SJ, et al. Optic nerve diffusion measurement from diffusion weighted imaging in optic neuritis. AJNR Am J Neuroradiol 2005;26:951–6.

32. Anand Trip S, Wheeler-Kingshott C, Jones SJ, et al. Optic nerve diffusion tensor imaging in optic neuritis. Neuroimage 2006;30:498–505.

33. Valsasina P, Rocca MA, Agosta F, et al. Mean diffusivity and fractional anisotropy histogram analysis of the cervical cord in MS patients. Neuroimage 2005;26:822–8.

34. Agosta F, Benedetti B, Rocca MA, et al. Quantification of cervical cord pathology in primary progressive MS using diffusion tensor MRI. Neurology 2005;64:631–5.

35. Hesseltine SM, Law M, Babb J, et al. Diffusion tensor imaging in multiple sclerosis: assessment of regional differences in the axial plane within normal-appearing cervical spinal cord. AJNR Am J Neuroradiol 2006;27:1189–93.

36. Benedetti B, Rovaris M, Pulizzi A, et al. A diffusion-tensor MRI study of the cervical cord damage in benign and secondary progressive MS patients. Neurology 2008;70(Suppl 1):A471.

37. Benedetti B, Valsasina P, Judica E, et al. Grading cervical cord damage in neuromyelitis optica and MS by diffusion tensor MRI. Neurology 2006;67: 161–3.

38. Ciccarelli O, Wheeler-Kingshott C, McLean MA, et al. Spinal cord spectroscopy and diffusion-based tractography to assess acute disability in multiple sclerosis. Brain 2007;130:2220–31.

39. Mori S, Kaufmann WE, Davatzikos C, et al. Imaging cortical association tracts in the human brain using diffusion-tensor-based axonal tracking. Magn Reson Med 2002;47:215–23.

40. Pagani E, Bammer R, Horsfield MA, et al. Diffusion MRI in multiple sclerosis: technical aspects and challenges. AJNR Am J Neuroradiol 2007;28: 411–20.

41. Pagani E, Filippi M, Rocca MA, et al. A method for obtaining tract-specific diffusion tensor MRI measurements in the presence of disease: application to patients with clinically isolated syndromes suggestive of multiple sclerosis. Neuroimage 2005; 26:258–65.

42. Wilson M, Tench CR, Morgan PS, et al. Pyramidal tract mapping by diffusion tensor magnetic resonance imaging in multiple sclerosis: improving correlations with disability. J Neurol Neurosurg Psychiatr 2003;74:203–7.

43. Lin X, Tench CR, Morgan PS, et al. Importance sampling in MS: use of diffusion tensor tractography to quantify pathology related to specific impairment. J Neurol Sci 2005;237:13–9.

44. Lin F, Yu C, Jiang T, et al. Diffusion tensor tractography-based group mapping of the pyramidal tract in relapsing-remitting multiple sclerosis patients. AJNR Am J Neuroradiol 2007;28:278–82.

45. Ciccarelli O, Toosy AT, Hickman SJ, et al. Optic radiation changes after optic neuritis detected by tractography-based group mapping. Hum Brain Mapp 2005;25:308–16.

46. Simon JH, Zhang S, Laidlaw DH, et al. Identification of fibers at risk for degeneration by diffusion tractography in patients at high risk for MS after a clinically isolated syndrome. J Mag Reson Imaging 2006;24:983–8.

47. Reich DS, Smith SA, Zackowski KM, et al. Multiparametric magnetic resonance imaging analysis of the corticospinal tract in multiple sclerosis. Neuroimage 2007;38:271–9.

48. Rocca MA, Pagani E, Absinta M, et al. Altered functional and structural connectivities in patients with MS: a 3-T study. Neurology 2007;69:2136–45.

49. Rocca MA, Valsasina P, Ceccarelli A, et al. Structural and functional MRI correlates of Stroop control in benign MS. Hum Brain Mapp 2007, in press.

50. Ashburner J, Friston KJ. Voxel-based morphometry-the methods. Neuroimage 2000;11:805–21.

51. Filippi M, Agosta F, Rocca MA. Regional assessment of brain atrophy: a novel approach to achieve a more complete picture of tissue damage associated with central nervous system disorders? AJNR Am J Neuroradiol 2007;28:255–9.

52. Ceccarelli A, Rocca MA, Pagani E, et al. The topographical distribution of tissue injury in benign MS: a 3T multiparametric study. Neuroimage 2008;39:1499–509.

53. Pagani E, Horsfield MA, Rocca MA, et al. Assessing atrophy of the major white matter fiber bundles of the brain from diffusion tensor MRI data. Magn Reson Med 2007;58:527–34.

54. Pagani E, Agosta F, Rocca MA, Caputo D, et al. Voxel-based analysis derived from fractional anisotropy images of white matter volume changes with aging. Neuroimage 2008;41:657–67.

55. Rosso C, Remy P, Creange A, et al. Diffusion-weighted MR imaging characteristics of an acute strokelike form of multiple sclerosis. AJNR Am J Neuroradiol 2006;27:1006–8.

56. Lin F, Yu C, Jiang T, et al. Discriminative analysis of relapsing neuromyelitis optica and relapsing-remitting multiple sclerosis based on two-dimensional histogram from diffusion tensor imaging. Neuroimage 2006;31:543–9.

57. Agosta F, Rocca MA, Benedetti B, et al. MR imaging assessment of brain and cervical cord damage in patients with neuroborreliosis. AJNR Am J Neuroradiol 2006;27:892–4.

58. Assaf Y, Chapman J, Ben-Bashat D, et al. White matter changes in multiple sclerosis: correlation of q-space diffusion MRI and ^{1}H MRS. Magn Reson Imaging 2005;23:703–10.

Proton Magnetic Resonance Spectroscopy in Multiple Sclerosis

Balasrinivasa R. Sajja, PhD[a], Jerry S. Wolinsky, MD[b],
Ponnada A. Narayana, PhD[c],*

KEYWORDS

- Proton magnetic resonance spectroscopy
- Multiple sclerosis • Brain metabolites

Conventional magnetic resonance (cMR) imaging is exquisitely sensitive in visualizing multiple sclerosis (MS) lesions in brain and spinal cord, but has limited pathologic specificity. Also, cMR imaging is limited in the detection of subtle, disease-related changes in the normal-appearing white matter (NAWM).[1] This limitation can be overcome to some extent by combining MR imaging with magnetic resonance spectroscopy (MRS), which allows detection of tissue biochemical changes for improved pathologic specificity. Because biochemical changes precede anatomic changes, MRS detects tissue pathologic changes even before the appearance of lesions on cMR imaging.[2] The unique biochemical information provided by MRS also complements the information from advanced MR imaging techniques, such as magnetization transfer (MT) and diffusion tensor (DT) MR imaging, in providing a more detailed and specific pathologic information. This information in turn allows us to follow MS disease evolution, better understand its pathogenesis, evaluate the disease severity, establish a prognosis, and objectively evaluate the efficacy of therapeutic interventions.[3–5]

This article is divided into three major sections: (1) brief introduction to MRS, (2) review of MRS and its application to MS lesions, NAWM, gray matter, and spinal cord, and (3) role of MRS in clinical trials. Because of the large number of publications on MRS in MS, wherever possible we have referenced more recent and relevant review articles.

MAGNETIC RESONANCE SPECTROSCOPY

In contrast to MR imaging, which mainly relies on the proton (^1H), MRS can be performed using various nuclei. Of all these nuclei, ^1H and ^{31}P are most commonly used for MRS studies. For several reasons, including sensitivity and hardware considerations, proton MRS (^1H-MRS) is the common choice for investigating neurologic disorders. ^1H-MRS provides access to a large number of biomolecules or metabolites, such as N-acetylaspartate (NAA; some authors refer to it as NA to acknowledge that the NAA peak has contributions from N-acetylaspartate and other N-acetyl moieties, such as N-acetyl aspartyl glutamate [NAAG]. In this article NA and NAA are used interchangeably.), choline (Cho), creatine (Cr), myoinositol (mI), glutamate (Glu), and glutamine (Gln), macromolecules, lipids, and lactate (Lac). The positions of metabolite peaks in the spectrum, expressed as parts per million (ppm), are independent of the magnetic field strength. NAA is an amino acid

This work was supported in part by NIH/NIBIB Grant No. EB02095.
a Department of Radiology, University of Nebraska Medical Center, 981045 Nebraska Medical Center, Omaha, NE 68198-1045, USA
b Department of Neurology, University of Texas Medical School at Houston, 6431 Fannin Street, Houston, TX 77030, USA
c Department of Diagnostic and Interventional Imaging, University of Texas Medical School at Houston, 6431 Fannin Street, Houston, TX 77030, USA
* Corresponding author.
E-mail address: ponnada.a.narayana@uth.tmc.edu (P.A. Narayana).

derivative synthesized in neurons and transported down axons and its main resonance appears at 2.02 ppm. NAA is generally believed to be a specific marker of neurons, axons, and dendrites.[6] On this basis, reduced NAA concentration is generally interpreted as neuronal/axonal dysfunction or loss. This interpretation has been confirmed by ^{1}H-MRS and histology studies on biopsied samples.[7] In general, Glu and Gln are not resolved well even at 3.0 T and combination of resonances from these two is commonly referred to as Glx. The resonances from Glx appear between 2.1 and 2.4 ppm. Although some studies have focused on the evaluation of the total Glu and Gln levels under pathologic conditions, other studies have used spectral editing methods to resolve the Glu resonance. Recently Hurd and colleagues[8] have used a modified conventional spectral localization technique in which data are collected over multiple echo times (TE). This method detects a single-line Glu resonance at 2.35 ppm. Srinivasan and colleagues[9] have shown elevated Glu concentrations in acute lesions ($P = .02$) and NAWM ($P = .03$), with no significant elevation in chronic lesions ($P = .77$) in patients who have MS compared with normal subjects. The primary resonance of Cr occurs at 3.0 ppm and has contributions from creatine and phosphocreatine. Elevated Cr levels may represent gliosis.[7] Cho signals at 3.2 ppm have contributions from multiple molecules that include phosphorylcholine, glycerophosphorylcholine, and choline plasmalogen, and a minor contribution from acetylcholine and choline.[10] Cho peak seems to reflect cell membrane metabolism.[3] Also, elevated Cho concentration represents heightened cell membrane turnover as seen in demyelination, remyelination, inflammation, and gliosis in patients who have MS.[3] mI exhibits two resonances at 3.5 ppm and 4.06 ppm. Because of its proximity to tissue water resonance, the amplitude of the 4.06-ppm peak is affected by the degree of water suppression and is not considered to be a reliable indicator of mI concentration. Brain osmolyte mI seems to be glia specific and it is not found in neurons.[11] Also, mI is a precursor of phospholipid membrane constituents, and its concentration is affected by the formation and breakdown of myelin. Lac is generally seen as a doublet that resonates at 1.33 ppm. It is the end product of anaerobic glycolysis and is not commonly observed in normal brain. It is increased in acute MS lesions and is related to macrophage activation after membrane breakdown. Lipids along with macromolecules (referred to as lipids for brevity) appear as broad peaks and resonate between 0.8 and 1.5 ppm. In healthy tissues, there should be weak lipid peaks in the spectrum unless contaminated by subcutaneous fat from nonneural tissues. These peaks have been reported in MS and are believed to represent demyelination/remyelination.[2] By measuring the concentration changes in brain metabolites, MRS has provided evidence of early pathology and myelin damage/repair in MS that is not evident on cMR imaging.[12,13]

Acquisition

^{1}H-MRS can be acquired with spatial information preserved (localized ^{1}H-MRS), as is most commonly done, or obtained from the whole brain by sacrificing spatial information.[14] Point resolved spectroscopy (PRESS)[15] and stimulated echo acquisition mode (STEAM)[16] are the two most commonly used localization techniques in ^{1}H-MRS. Spectral contamination from extrameningeal tissues is minimized by suppressing the signals from the outer volume.[17] **Fig. 1** demonstrates the placement of eight outer volume suppression bands. The PRESS localization provides better signal-to-noise ratio (SNR) compared with STEAM technique. STEAM allows shorter TE than PRESS, however.

Localized ^{1}H-MRS is acquired in either a single-voxel or multivoxel mode. In single-voxel MRS, spectral data are acquired from one location at a time. The volume of this region is typically 1 to 8 cm^3. This approach involves shorter acquisition and processing times. High-quality spectrum is relatively easy to acquire in this mode. Multivoxel mode, also referred to as ^{1}H-MRS imaging or chemical shift imaging, allows simultaneous acquisition of ^{1}H-MRS data from multiple voxels and allows mapping regional distribution of metabolite concentrations and generating metabolic images. Multivoxel MRS can be acquired in two dimensions or three dimensions (3D) and generally offers superior spatial resolution (<1 cm^3) compared with single voxel. Generally, ^{1}H-MRS imaging is acquired from a volume that is prelocalized using either PRESS or STEAM. It is also possible to acquire ^{1}H-MRS imaging without any prior volume or slab localization (see, for example, Sharma and colleagues.)[18] ^{1}H-MRS imaging involves relatively long acquisition times, which, however, can be considerably shortened by reduced k-space encoding.[19] One way of accelerating ^{1}H-MRS imaging acquisition is to use fast spectral-spatial encoding by using echo-planar (EP)–based techniques.[20,21] With multislice and multiecho sequences, it is possible to acquire spectra from whole brain[21] within reasonable scan times. Combining EPI-based techniques with recent advances in parallel MR imaging,

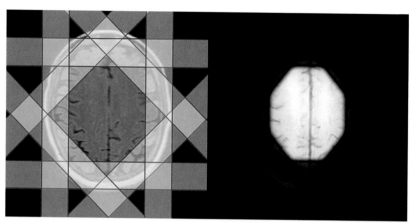

Fig. 1. Application of outer volume suppression bands to minimize extrameningeal tissue contamination. (*Left*) Eight outer volume suppression bands on one of the five images (each, 3-mm thickness) that represent the spectroscopic volume of interest (15-mm thickness). (*Right*) Localized image (15-mm slice thickness with the application of the suppression bands) from which ¹H-MRS imaging is acquired.

such as sensitivity encoding (SENSE)[22] or generalized autocalibrating partially parallel acquisitions (GRAPPA)[23] with radiofrequency (RF) coil arrays can further accelerate ¹H-MRS imaging data acquisition.[24–26] The data acquired with these approaches generally suffer from reduced SNR, however. Determination of absolute metabolite concentration is also somewhat problematic with parallel acquisition schemes.

¹H-MRS can be acquired at either long or short TE. Long TE ¹H-MRS provides a well-defined baseline by suppressing peaks arising from short T2 metabolites, such as lipids and macromolecules, and makes spectral quantification simpler and more robust. Long TE ¹H-MRS may be preferable if the interest is in the detection of the three major resonances: NAA, Cr, and Cho. Because of their relatively short T2 relaxation times, signals from metabolites, such as Glx, lipids, macromolecules, and other myelin breakdown products, can be detected only at short TE. Even though the broad spectral baseline in short TE ¹H-MRS makes the spectral quantification more difficult, this approach has the potential to provide important information about altered tissue biochemistry that may not be available at long TE.[4] There is an increasing interest in short TE ¹H-MRS imaging for visualizing short T2 metabolites, which should result in improved pathologic characterization of tissues.[3] As an example, single voxel spectra acquired at 3 T with short and long TE, with signal mostly localized to white matter of normal brain, are shown in **Fig. 2**.

The macromolecular and lipid resonances exhibit significant overlap with the other metabolites. By nulling the metabolite resonances with an inversion recovery sequence, it is possible to improve the detection of these short TE resonances. This method was used by Mader and colleagues[27] for separating lipids from other metabolites in acute MS lesions.

Although localized techniques can be used to acquire spectra from the volume of interest (VOI), nonlocalized sequence can provide MRS from the entire head. The strong broad lipid signals arising from non-brain tissues obscure the resonances from other metabolites. By subtracting

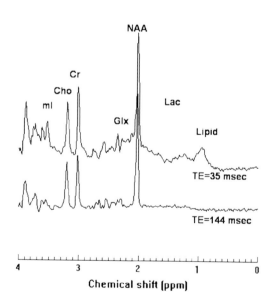

Fig. 2. Single voxel spectra with short TE (35 milliseconds) and long TE (144 milliseconds) acquired from white matter region of a normal brain at 3.0 Tesla. The large number of metabolite peaks with broad baseline can be observed in the short TE spectrum (*top*). In contrast, long TE spectrum (*bottom*) has relatively flat baseline and fewer metabolite peaks.

the data acquired with and without NAA nulling (through an inversion recovery sequence), however, it is possible to remove/minimize strong lipid signals and visualize resonances from other metabolites.[14] Because NAA is restricted to neurons/axons, it is implicitly localized to brain. The presence of other resonances in non-brain tissues compromises the quantification of metabolites such as Cr. This approach is thus reliable only when quantifying the whole-brain NAA (WBNAA) concentration.[14] Because of severe magnetic field inhomogeneities present at air-tissue interfaces this technique captures about 90% of the NAA signal intensity in the brain.[28] Although WBNAA measurements do not provide any information about the spatial distribution of metabolite concentrations, this approach eliminates image registration problems from scan to scan in serial studies. The reproducibility of WBNAA levels across institutions and MR scanners and field strengths has been shown to be satisfactory.[29] WBNAA measurements can be used to quantify the global neuronal and axonal injury to monitor the effect of neuroprotective agents in MS.[30]

Quantification

The inherently quantitative nature of MRS allows objective monitoring of disease state and response to therapeutic intervention. This monitoring requires accurate spectral quantification, however. Expressing the metabolite levels as a ratio relative to Cr is one of the most common and simplest ways of spectral quantification. The interpretation of the metabolite ratios becomes equivocal, however, if the concentration of Cr varies with pathology.[2] In addition, representing brain metabolite concentrations as ratios does not provide complete information and could lead to significant errors.[31,32] Absolute quantification of metabolite concentrations is therefore highly desirable for proper interpretation of the MRS data. Nevertheless the NAA/Cr ratio is commonly used in MS.[33] Among the methods for estimating the absolute metabolite concentrations, use of internal water as a standard has been shown to provide acceptable accuracy and interlaboratory reproducibility.[2,34] This method depends on knowledge of water distribution and relaxation times in different tissues, however. Absolute concentrations can also be measured using the LCModel.[35] This method analyzes the in vivo spectrum as a linear combination of spectra from individual metabolites contained in a solution (model spectrum). The model spectrum is acquired using the same sequence as that used for in vivo spectra and provides the maximum prior knowledge for the

spectral analysis. LCModel uses a nearly model-free constrained regularization method that automatically accounts for the fitted baseline and spectral lineshape to be consistent with the data.[36]

Usually, the ¹H-MRS imaging quantification procedures involve extensive computational time, and in some cases, significant human intervention. Currently, the most commonly used quantification methods are based on line fitting using nonlinear least squares optimization, such as the Levenberg-Marquardt algorithm.[35,37–39] The relatively long computational time becomes even more problematic when considering 3D ¹H-MRS imaging and scans from multicenter clinical trials wherein a large amount of data needs to be processed. For ¹H-MRS imaging to become a routine clinical tool, complete automation of quantification procedures and reduction of processing times close to real time are necessary. The processing time could be reduced by using a high-performance computing environment. This process is expensive, involves development of complicated algorithms, and is not an option in routine laboratory/clinical settings. Another approach is to develop fast methods, such as those based on artificial neural networks (ANN). ANN has been used to develop automated methods to quantify ¹H-MRS data.[40,41] These techniques are limited to either single-voxel ¹H-MRS or magnitude spectral data acquired at long TE using lineshapes that may not be completely appropriate.[42] Recently, Bhat and colleagues[43] have used radial basis function neural networks to demonstrate the feasibility of quantifying short TE, phased ¹H-MRS imaging. This method is limited to ratios, however, and thus does not allow absolute concentrations to be measured.

Several excellent software packages, both free and commercial, are available for spectral quantification. The most commonly used analysis packages include LCModel,[35] jMRUI,[44] and MIDAS.[45] Most of these packages involve minimal human intervention and are capable of providing absolute concentrations, but involve long processing times. Different analysis methods and their strengths and weaknesses in computing absolute brain metabolite concentrations were recently reviewed.[31]

Because of relatively large spectroscopic voxels, spectra have contributions from different types of brain tissues, particularly cerebrospinal fluid (CSF). For accurate estimation of metabolite concentrations, it is important to determine the relative volumes of each tissue that contributes to a given spectroscopic voxel. This estimation requires combining the MRS imaging data with tissue segmentation, based on the high-resolution MR imaging data.[37]

APPLICATION OF MAGNETIC RESONANCE SPECTROSCOPY TO MULTIPLE SCLEROSIS
Lesions

There is a general consensus that chronic MS lesions exhibit reduced NAA levels, indicating neuronal/axonal loss. This observation is particularly true in those lesions that also appear hypointense on T1-weighted images (also commonly referred to as "black holes").[46] In one study, metabolite concentrations from chronic lesions of patients who had relapsing-remitting (RR)MS (n = 9), secondary progressive (SP)MS (n = 10), primary progressive (PP)MS (n = 6), and benign MS (BMS) (n = 5) were measured and compared with those from white matter of a normal control group (n = 9).[47] A highly significant reduction in NA (the sum of NAA and NAAG) was found in patients who had RRMS, PPMS, and SPMS compared with controls. In patients who had BMS, however, there was no significant difference in NA compared with controls. A significant inverse correlation between NA from lesions in patients who had MS and disability was observed (r = -0.364, .05>P>.02).[47] Increased Cr and Cho levels were also observed in lesions, suggesting (1) ongoing gliosis and remyelination in isointense lesions on T1-weighted MR images, and (2) membrane turnover (de- and remyelination).[48]

Acute MS lesions, as detected by gadolinium (Gd) enhancement, demonstrate a range of abnormalities on ¹H-MRS. These abnormalities include reduced NAA, increased Cho, and presence of lipids.[2,49–52] Histopathology on biopsied brain tissues demonstrates reduced NAA levels even in the acute phase of the disease;[53] this could be the result of axonal loss or reflect reversible axonal dysfunction attributable to functional impairment.[52,54–56] Accordingly, serial MR imaging (with Gd administration) and ¹H-MRS imaging studies showed transient changes in NAA levels in some acute lesions, which recovered with time.[2] Narayana and colleagues[2] have observed that metabolite levels, including NAA, reach their minimum value when lesion volume reaches its maximum. This observation suggests that the observed decrease in metabolite concentrations, at least partially, can be attributed to presence of edema within the lesions and is not solely to compromised tissue metabolism. Cho levels are shown to increase in acute MS lesions,[2,51,57] in addition to Lac and mI resonance intensities.[52,58] The presence of lipids in some, but not all, lesions was reported in RRMS subjects by Narayana and colleagues,[2] suggesting the presence of active demyelination/remyelination.

Normal-Appearing White Matter

It is now generally agreed, based on MRS,[3,12] MT,[59] and DTI[60] studies, that the NAWM in patients who have MS is abnormal. By exploiting the large spatial coverage allowed by multivoxel ¹H-MRS, it has been demonstrated that metabolic abnormalities in patients who have MS are more diffuse and are not restricted to lesion sites alone.[2,37,48,61–64] ¹H-MRS studies have clearly demonstrated reduced NAA levels in NAWM, suggesting axonal/neuronal loss/dysfunction as the underlying pathologic substrate. The reduced NAA levels on ¹H-MRS have been confirmed by histopathology as secondary to axonal loss.[7,65] In serial ¹H-MRS studies, increased Cho and lipid levels were observed from NAWM regions that subsequently went on to develop MR imaging–visible lesions.[2,66] These observations are consistent with MR imaging studies that showed alterations in MT ratio (MTR) values before appearance of macroscopic lesions on MR imaging.[67] In addition, based on increased mI,[68] Cr, and Cho levels, increased cellularity (gliosis, inflammation) was also postulated to occur in NAWM of patients who have MS.[48]

In a preliminary study, annual MRS imaging was acquired for 2 years from 20 patients and 10 healthy controls to characterize the metabolite changes in early RRMS.[69] The concentrations of NAA, Cr, Cho, mI, and Glx were estimated in NAWM and cortical gray matter (cGM). At baseline, the concentration of NAA was 7% lower in NAWM of patients who had MS compared with the control group and 8.7% lower in cGM. Tissue metabolite profiles did not significantly change in subjects who had MS nor did they differ between subjects who had MS and healthy controls, with the exception of NAA concentrations that tended to recover from baseline. This study suggests that in the early phases of the disease the neuronal/axonal damage may be at least partially reversible. Leary and colleagues[70] have performed single-voxel ¹H-MRS of NAWM in PPMS (n = 24) patients and in 16 age-matched controls. NAA/Cr was significantly lower in NAWM from patients than in the white matter from controls, suggesting that axonal loss occurs in NAWM in patients who have PPMS and may well be a factor associated with disease progression in this disease phenotype. No significant difference was observed in Cr concentration between patients and controls. A multicenter ¹H-MRS imaging study of 40 patients who had PPMS showed significantly lower NAA/Cr compared with healthy volunteers, but no significant difference between lesions and NAWM was observed.[33] Twenty-four of these patients had evident lipid peaks in nonlesion brain tissue locations. **Fig. 3** shows, as an example, the presence of strong lipid peaks in the spectra from normal appearing brain tissue of a patient who had PPMS. In another study, metabolite concentrations were obtained with 3D MRS and the VOI centered on the corpus callosum in 11 patients who had RRMS and 9 controls.[71] In NAWM, the concentration of NAA was observed to be 9% lower in patients compared with controls. The

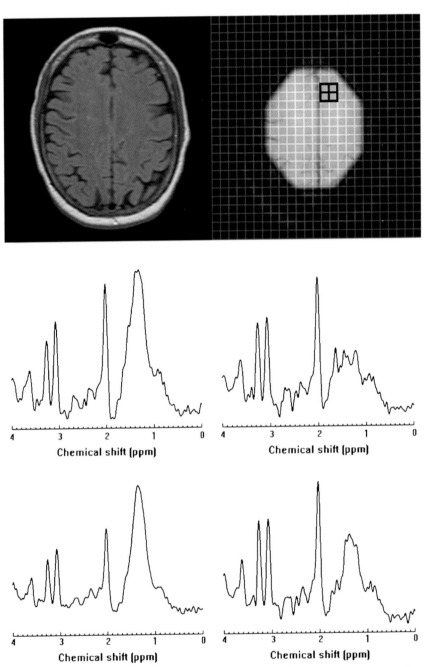

Fig. 3. Lipid peaks in normal-appearing tissue of a patient who had primary progressive multiple sclerosis. (*Top left*) One of the five MR images (each 3-mm thick) of the cross section of the brain location from where the ¹H-MRS imaging data were acquired. (*Right*) Collapsed image representing the spectroscopic volume of interest (thickness, 15 mm). The small grid on the collapsed image represents the spatial location of spectra shown in the bottom panel. Strong lipid peaks can be observed in these spectra. The spectra were acquired at TE of 30 ms.

same study showed an increase in Cr and Cho by 22% and 32%, respectively. These elevated Cho levels differentiated patients from controls with 100% specificity and greater than 90% sensitivity.

Suhy and colleagues[72] compared metabolite levels in patients who had PPMS (n = 15) and RRMS (n = 13) with those of controls (n = 20). Cr in NAWM of patients who had PPMS was higher compared with controls (P = .035) and patients who had RRMS (P = .038). Also, Cr increased in focal lesions from PPMS compared with lesions from RRMS (P = .044) and compared with control white matter (P = .041). NAA was similarly reduced in NAWM from PPMS and RRMS compared with controls. The increased Cr in NAWM in PPMS relative to RRMS is consistent with the notion that the progressive disability in PPMS may be associated with gliosis and axonal loss, whereas disability in RRMS may be secondary to an increased burden of acute inflammatory lesions and axonal loss.[72]

Data on NAWM in clinically isolated syndrome (CIS) are limited. In 14 of 42 patients who had a single acute episode of optic neuritis, Tourbah and colleagues[73] reported decreased NAA, increased Cho, and the presence of lipids. In 96 patients who had CIS suggestive of MS, Fernando and colleagues[74] reported increased concentration of mI relative to controls, a finding suggestive for the presence of gliosis. No significant difference in other metabolites was observed. In a prospective study on patients who had CIS suggestive of MS, Wattjes and colleagues[75,76] studied 31 patients and 20 controls. These authors observed 8.1% decrease in NAA (P = .012) in the NAWM of patients relative to controls. Changes in Cr, Cho, and mI were not observed.

Gray Matter

Cortical pathology in MS is well recognized.[77,78] For several reasons GM lesions are difficult to visualize on MR imaging. Using advanced pulse sequences, such as double inversion recovery[79,80] and phase-sensitive inversion recovery sequence, it is possible to visualize some, but not all, cortical lesions.[81,82] Involvement of GM has been demonstrated by MTR,[83] DTI,[84,85] and ¹H-MRS studies.[18,68,86,87]

¹H-MRS of cGM is technically challenging because of its proximity to CSF and partial volume averaging from white matter.[88] In addition, many of the MRS studies that use outer volume suppression bands for minimizing contributions from non-neural tissues make it difficult to acquire MRS from the cGM that is close to the outer surface of the brain (see **Fig. 1**). Despite these limitations, MRS studies of cGM have been reported by a few

groups. For example, Sharma and colleagues,[18] by combining a double inversion recovery sequence in which both CSF and white matter were suppressed, demonstrated abnormalities in the cGM close to the midline fissure in patients who had MS using MRS imaging. By combining MRS imaging with image segmentation, this study has minimized contributions from WM and CSF to the VOI and showed in 52 patients who had RRMS marked lipid peaks arising from the normal-appearing GM, consistent with the presence of active demyelination/remyelination. No significant changes in major metabolite concentrations were observed compared with controls, however, suggesting no significant neuronal loss. The lack of significant changes of metabolites in cGM is consistent with another more recent report.[89]

Using short TE MRS imaging in 16 patients who had RRMS with short disease duration (mean disease duration of 1.8 years; range 0.6–2.8 years), Kapellar and colleagues[86] reported lower NAA (P = .01) and mI (P = .04) in cGM relative to controls. The reduced NAA in cGM suggested mild, but widespread, neuronal dysfunction or loss early on in the course of the disease.[86] In another study from the same group of 24 clinically early (median Expanded Disability Status Scale [EDSS] 1.2; range 0.0–3.0) patients who had RRMS, Chard and colleagues[68] reported significantly reduced NAA, Cho, and Glx. They also observed significant correlations between MS functional composite scores and the metabolite concentrations in cGM: Cr (r(s) = 0.524, P = .009), Glx (r(s) = 0.580, P = .003). No correlation was observed between clinical disability and the level of NAA, suggesting that reduced NAA reflects neuronal dysfunction, rather than neuronal loss, early on in RRMS.

GM NAA deficits were found in the progressive form of disease, which, however, did not significantly correlate with EDSS.[90] In another study, absolute concentrations of NAA, Cr, and Cho were measured in the occipital-parietal cortex of patients who had RRMS (n = 15) and SPMS (n = 15) and healthy subjects (n = 8).[91] Significantly lower values of NAA, Cr, and NAA/Cr ratio were detected in patients who had SPMS than in those who had RRMS and control subjects (P<.01), suggesting that the pathologic process in MS extends into cGM, particularly in the progressive form of the disease. Similar observations were reported in a more recent study on a small MS cohort.[87]

The levels of metabolites in the early stage of the disease seem to depend on lesion activity. In CIS suggestive of MS, Au Duong and colleagues[88] reported that the metabolite levels in GM are associated with the presence of enhancing lesions: when absent, there was no statistically significant difference in the GM metabolite levels between patients and controls; when present, a relative decrease in NAA level and an increase in Cho level were observed. This finding suggests that metabolite alterations seen in the GM in the early phase of the disease may be secondary to the inflammatory process, rather than to primary neuronal dysfunction.

MS also affects deep GM structures.[92,93] ^{1}H-MRS studies of the thalami were performed in patients who had RRMS (n = 14) and age-matched healthy controls (n = 14). Average NAA concentration in the thalami of patients who had RRMS was approximately 11% lower relative to controls ($P<.05$). In addition, about 25% lower mean normalized thalamic volumes were observed in patients compared with controls ($P<.005$). Decreases in thalamic NAA concentrations strongly correlated with thalamic volume loss.[94] The reduction of NAA concentration and thalamic volume suggests a neurodegenerative component to MS that is increasingly recognized in the disease.[95]

WHOLE BRAIN N-ACETYLASPARTATE

Recently, WBNAA as a marker of overall axonal/neuronal loss in the brain has been proposed.[96] The concentration levels of WBNAA and normalized brain volumes were significantly lower in patients who had PPMS than in healthy controls.[97] Also, WBNAA values and normalized brain volumes were not related, suggesting that MRS and atrophy assessment may provide complementary information about the extent of brain damage in PPMS. Axonal/neuronal damage in patients who have PPMS seems to occur, at least partially, independent of the burden of MR imaging–visible lesions.[97] In another study, WBNAA levels were compared with atrophy as a function of disease duration in a cohort of 42 patients who had RRMS. WBNAA levels were found to decrease 3.6 times faster than atrophy, suggesting that neuronal/axonal dysfunction precedes atrophy,[98] and that WBNAA may be a more sensitive indicator of disease progression than lesion load or atrophy.

Although axonal pathology has been known to occur in MS, it is less clear how early in the course of disease axonal damage starts to appear, or what its relation is to MR imaging–visible lesion load. To assess this early axonal pathology, Filippi and colleagues[99] estimated the WBNAA levels in 31 patients who had CIS suggestive of MS. The mean WBNAA concentration was significantly lower in patients compared with the controls.

It was not significantly different between patients who had or did not have enhancing lesions at baseline MR imaging or between patients who had or did not have lesion dissemination in time. WBNAA concentrations and lesion volumes were not correlated. These findings, consistent with histology and localized ^{1}H-MRS studies, suggest the presence of widespread axonal pathology in the earliest clinically symptomatic stage of MS.

SPINAL CORD

Involvement of spinal cord in MS and its potential role in patient disability has been recognized for some time.[100,101] Postmortem examination of patients who had MS reported substantial atrophy and axonal loss in the lateral columns at C3 and T2.[102] Cord atrophy and total axonal number are not strongly correlated, however,[103] suggesting that cord atrophy may underestimate axonal loss and may not provide a valid marker of disease progression.[104] ^{1}H-MRS may provide valuable information about true axonal damage in spinal cord in patients who have MS. In vivo ^{1}H-MRS of spinal cord is challenging because of magnetic field inhomogeneities around the cord, physiologic movements, and small cross-sectional size. It is not surprising, therefore, that relatively few ^{1}H-MRS studies of the spinal cord have been performed. Marliani and colleagues[105] demonstrated the feasibility of performing quantitative MRS in the cervical region on a clinical 3 T system.

^{1}H-MRS of normal-appearing spinal cord in patients who had MS showed significantly reduced NAA and altered concentration levels of other metabolites compared with healthy controls.[106] In one study, MRS was used to investigate the degree of neuronal damage in the cervical cord in patients who had MS. Spectra were acquired from spinal cord and brain in 11 patients and 11 controls. A 32% reduction of NAA concentration was observed in patients relative to controls ($P<.05$), indicating significant neuronal/axonal injury. Additionally, significant cord atrophy was observed in patients who had MS (15%, $P<.001$). No correlations between clinical measures and cord atrophy or brain lesion volume were found; however, spinal cord NAA correlated with the cerebellar subscore of the EDSS ($P<.005$). ^{1}H-MRS demonstrated cellular damage within the cord over and above the tissue atrophy seen on MR imaging.[104]

In another study, Ciccarelli and colleagues[107] acquired single-voxel ^{1}H-MRS from the cervical cord of 14 patients who had at least one lesion between C1 and C3. Thirteen age- and sex-matched control subjects were included in the study. Patients showed reduced NAA relative to controls. In patients, significant correlations between (1) EDSS and mI, Cho, Cr, and (2) 9-hole peg test (9-HPT) and Cr were observed. The concentration of mI was independently associated with the EDSS, whereas Cr and NAA were independently associated with the 9-HPT. Although the limited ¹H-MRS studies on cervical cord have provided useful information about tissue damage, the full potential of ¹H-MRS in spinal cord in patients who have MS has yet to be exploited.

EVALUATION OF TREATMENT EFFICACY

Immunomodulatory therapies, including glatiramer acetate (GA), interferon (IFN)-β, and natalizumab, are shown to be effective in reducing MR imaging–measured disease activity.[108–111] Because of its inherent quantitative nature, MRS is ideally suited for evaluating the efficacy of treatment. The effect of immunomodulatory treatments on brain metabolites for evaluating treatment efficacy was studied in multiple, but small, patient groups. In an open-label, nonrandomized pilot study of GA treatment in 15 patients who had RRMS, Narayanan and colleagues[112] measured NAA/Cr in a large VOI centered in the corpus callosum before treatment and 1 year after. The untreated and treated groups had similar mean baseline NAA/Cr and EDSS. At 1 year, the GA-treated group showed no change in the NAA/Cr ratio. The untreated group had a small (3.5%) but significant ($P = .015$) reduction in NAA/Cr. During this short period of treatment, GA was shown to stabilize the levels of brain NAA, which is consistent with the putative neuroprotective effect of the drug, GA.

In another pilot study, Khan and colleagues[109] obtained ¹H-MRS from 18 patients who had RRMS before and after treatment with GA. These patients were followed annually for 2 years. A small group of 4 treatment-naïve patients who had RRMS was also studied. ¹H-MRS imaging was acquired from a large VOI that contained both corpus callosum and adjacent white matter. The VOI included both lesions and NAWM. The mean NAA/Cr was measured from the whole VOI and NAWM. After 2 years, NAA/Cr in the GA-treated group increased significantly (10.7%) in the VOI, and by 7.1% in the NAWM. In the untreated group, NAA/Cr decreased by 8.9% at 2 years in the VOI and 8.2% in the NAWM. This study showed that treatment with GA may lead to axonal metabolic recovery and protection from sublethal axonal injury in patients who have RRMS. Long-term results of this ongoing study after 4 years of annual brain MRS examinations were reported recently.[113] Compared with baseline, at year 4, patients receiving continuous GA therapy showed an overall increase of 12.7% in NAA/Cr ($P = .03$) within the entire VOI and by 9.6% ($P = .04$) in the NAWM. Three patients in the control group who began therapy with GA during the course of the study showed similar increases in NAA/Cr after the first year of therapy. These data support the notion of a possible sustained effect of GA in RRMS and the feasibility of using MRS in long-term investigative studies of MS.[113]

In a multicenter longitudinal MRS imaging study, the efficacy of GA treatment in 58 patients who had PPMS was investigated annually for 3 years.[114] This patient population was a subcohort of the PROMiSe trial patients.[115] Quantitative NAA/Cr and Cho/Cr were compared between GA-treated and placebo-treated patients who had PPMS. This study failed to demonstrate a significant effect of GA on the metabolite concentrations. There were no significant changes in metabolite concentrations in untreated patients who had PPMS over 3 years. These findings are different from those in RRMS described earlier in this article and may suggest that substantive decreases in NAA/Cr may have occurred at an earlier stage of disease in PPMS and treatment with GA may not result in improvement of the metabolite profile.[114]

Longitudinal MRS studies have been performed in 10 patients who had RRMS who, after baseline examination, received IFNβ-1b. Spectra were acquired up to 34 months at different time points (from 8–20 time points), and absolute concentrations of NAA, Cr, and Cho were determined in a large nonenhancing lesion and contralateral NAWM.[116] The concentrations of Cho and Cr were found to be higher in MS than in healthy controls.[116] These studies, except in 1 out of 10 patients, failed to demonstrate any effect of IFNβ-1b on the metabolic levels.

¹H-MRS has also been used to investigate the modifications of brain metabolites in the initial phase of IFNβ-1a treatment.[117] This study was performed on 5 patients who had RRMS who were treated with intramuscular IFNβ-1a for 6 months and 5 untreated patients. Patients were evaluated at the beginning of the study and in the first, third, and sixth month of treatment. In white matter lesions, NAA, Cho, Cr, and mI peaks did not vary significantly over the entire period of study in the untreated group. In the treated group, there was a significant increase in Cho at the first month relative to the pretreatment period that continued to increase at months 3 and 6 ($P<.001$). A slight but not statistically significant increase in Cho was also found in the NAWM from the patients treated with IFNβ-1a.

In a small pilot study, ^{1}H-MRS was performed in 10 patients who had RRMS before and after 1 year of treatment with subcutaneous IFNβ-1b. NAA/Cr was measured in a large central brain volume.[118] These measurements were compared with those from 6 untreated patients selected for similar range of EDSS scores and mean NAA/Cr at baseline. NAA/Cr in the treated group showed an increase of 5.5% at 12 months of therapy, whereas this ratio decreased in the untreated group, but not significantly. NAA/Cr was significantly higher in the treated group at 12 months than in the untreated group,[118] suggesting an effect of IFNβ-1b in restoring neural integrity.

Unfortunately, many of these studies are based on small patient populations followed over short intervals. Lack of standardized acquisition and analysis protocols makes it difficult to evaluate the results critically.

SUMMARY

^{1}H-MRS is a valuable tool that could contribute to objectively following the evolution of MS to the understanding of its pathogenesis, evaluating disease severity, establishing prognosis, and assessing the efficacy of therapeutic interventions. Some of the most compelling evidence that axonal loss is a major cause of disability in MS has come from ^{1}H-MRS studies that show reduced NAA levels in brains of these patients. ^{1}H-MRS studies have shown that axonal damage is an early event that occurs before the formation of MR imaging–visible lesions. Several technical factors that include poor SNR, long acquisition times, poor spatial resolution, limited spatial coverage, and complex data processing have so far limited the use of ^{1}H-MRS in routine clinical practice. Recent developments of high-field MR imaging scanners for improved SNR and spectral resolution, introduction of parallel imaging, fast analysis techniques, and the availability of free analysis tools should greatly facilitate a more widespread use of ^{1}H-MRS in the diagnosis and management of MS. Another aspect of MRS that needs to be addressed is the standardization of acquisition and analysis protocols. A first step toward achieving the standardization, based on single-voxel MRS, has recently been proposed.[13] Although this is an appropriate first step, standardized protocols that include multivoxel MRS for increased spatial coverage and exploit the full potential of MR hardware and software are needed.

REFERENCES

1. Rovaris M, Comi G, Filippi M. The role of non-conventional MR techniques to study multiple sclerosis patients. J Neurol Sci 2001;186(Suppl 1):S3–9.

2. Narayana PA, Doyle TJ, Lai D, et al. Serial proton magnetic resonance spectroscopic imaging, contrast-enhanced magnetic resonance imaging, and quantitative lesion volumetry in multiple sclerosis. Ann Neurol 1998;43(1):56–71.

3. Narayana PA. Magnetic resonance spectroscopy in the monitoring of multiple sclerosis. J Neuroimaging 2005;15(4 Suppl):46S–57S.

4. Wolinsky JS, Narayana PA. Magnetic resonance spectroscopy in multiple sclerosis: window into the diseased brain. Curr Opin Neurol 2002;15(3): 247–51.

5. Gonzalez-Toledo E, Kelley RE, Minagar A. Role of magnetic resonance spectroscopy in diagnosis and management of multiple sclerosis. Neurol Res 2006;28(3):280–3.

6. Lin A, Ross BD, Harris K, et al. Efficacy of proton magnetic resonance spectroscopy in neurological diagnosis and neurotherapeutic decision making. NeuroRx 2005;2(2):197–214.

7. Bitsch A, Bruhn H, Vougioukas V, et al. Inflammatory CNS demyelination: histopathologic correlation with in vivo quantitative proton MR spectroscopy. AJNR Am J Neuroradiol 1999;20(9):1619–27.

8. Hurd R, Sailasuta N, Srinivasan R, et al. Measurement of brain glutamate using TE-averaged PRESS at 3 T. Magn Reson Med 2004;51(3):435–40.

9. Srinivasan R, Sailasuta N, Hurd R, et al. Evidence of elevated glutamate in multiple sclerosis using magnetic resonance spectroscopy at 3 T. Brain 2005; 128(Pt 5):1016–25.

10. Frahm J, Hanefeld F. Localized proton magnetic resonance spectroscopy of brain disorders in childhood. In: Bachelard HS, editor, Advances in neurochemistry. vol. 18. New York: Plenum; 1997. p. 329–402.

11. Brand A, Richter-Landsberg C, Leibfritz D. Multinuclear NMR studies on the energy metabolism of glial and neuronal cells. Dev Neurosci 1993; 15(3–5):289–98.

12. De Stefano N, Filippi M. MR spectroscopy in multiple sclerosis. J Neuroimaging 2007;17(Suppl 1): 31S–5S.

13. De Stefano N, Filippi M, Miller D, et al. Guidelines for using proton MR spectroscopy in multicenter clinical MS studies. Neurology 2007;69(20): 1942–52.

14. Gonen O, Viswanathan AK, Catalaa I, et al. Total brain N-acetylaspartate concentration in normal, age-grouped females: quantitation with non-echo proton NMR spectroscopy. Magn Reson Med 1998;40(5):684–9.

15. Bottomley PA. Spatial localization in NMR spectroscopy in vivo. Ann N Y Acad Sci 1987;508:333–48.

16. Frahm J, Merboldt K-D, Hanicke W. Localized proton spectroscopy using stimulated echoes. J Magn Reson 1987;72(3):502–8.

17. Posse S, DeCarli C, Le Bihan D. Three-dimensional echo-planar MR spectroscopic imaging at short echo times in the human brain. Radiology 1994; 192(3):733–8.

18. Sharma R, Narayana PA, Wolinsky JS. Grey matter abnormalities in multiple sclerosis: proton magnetic resonance spectroscopic imaging. Mult Scler 2001;7(4):221–6.

19. Maudsley AA, Matson GB, Hugg JW, et al. Reduced phase encoding in spectroscopic imaging. Magn Reson Med 1994;31(6):645–51.

20. Posse S, Tedeschi G, Risinger R, et al. High speed 1H spectroscopic imaging in human brain by echo planar spatial-spectral encoding. Magn Reson Med 1995;33(1):34–40.

21. Mathiesen HK, Tscherning T, Sorensen PS, et al. Multi-slice echo-planar spectroscopic MR imaging provides both global and local metabolite measures in multiple sclerosis. Magn Reson Med 2005;53(4):750–9.

22. Pruessmann KP, Weiger M, Scheidegger MB, et al. SENSE: sensitivity encoding for fast MRI. Magn Reson Med 1999;42(5):952–62.

23. Griswold MA, Jakob PM, Heidemann RM, et al. Generalized autocalibrating partially parallel acquisitions (GRAPPA). Magn Reson Med 2002;47(6): 1202–10.

24. Lin FH, Tsai SY, Otazo R, et al. Sensitivity-encoded (SENSE) proton echo-planar spectroscopic imaging (PEPSI) in the human brain. Magn Reson Med 2007;57(2):249–57.

25. Tsai SY, Otazo R, Posse S, et al. Accelerated proton echo planar spectroscopic imaging (PEPSI) using GRAPPA with a 32-channel phased-array coil. Magn Reson Med 2008;59(5):989–98.

26. Otazo R, Tsai SY, Lin FH, et al. Accelerated short-TE 3D proton echo-planar spectroscopic imaging using 2D-SENSE with a 32-channel array coil. Magn Reson Med 2007;58(6):1107–16.

27. Mader I, Seeger U, Weissert R, et al. Proton MR spectroscopy with metabolite-nulling reveals elevated macromolecules in acute multiple sclerosis. Brain 2001;124(Pt 5):953–61.

28. Gonen O, Grossman RI. The accuracy of whole brain N-acetylaspartate quantification. Magn Reson Imaging 2000;18(10):1255–8.

29. Benedetti B, Rigotti DJ, Liu S, et al. Reproducibility of the whole-brain N-acetylaspartate level across institutions, MR scanners, and field strengths. AJNR Am J Neuroradiol 2007;28(1):72–5.

30. Rigotti DJ, Inglese M, Gonen O. Whole-brain N-acetylaspartate as a surrogate marker of neuronal damage in diffuse neurologic disorders. AJNR Am J Neuroradiol 2007;28(10):1843–9.

31. Jansen JF, Backes WH, Nicolay K, et al. 1H MR spectroscopy of the brain: absolute quantification of metabolites. Radiology 2006;240(2):318–32.

32. Li BS, Wang H, Gonen O. Metabolite ratios to assumed stable creatine level may confound the quantification of proton brain MR spectroscopy. Magn Reson Imaging 2003;21(8):923–8.

33. Narayana PA, Wolinsky JS, Rao SB, et al. Multi-centre proton magnetic resonance spectroscopy imaging of primary progressive multiple sclerosis. Mult Scler 2004;10(Suppl 1):S73–8.

34. Keevil SF, Barbiroli B, Brooks JC, et al. Absolute metabolite quantification by in vivo NMR spectroscopy: II. a multicentre trial of protocols for in vivo localised proton studies of human brain. Magn Reson Imaging 1998;16(9):1093–106.

35. Provencher SW. Estimation of metabolite concentrations from localized in vivo proton NMR spectra. Magn Reson Med 1993;30(6):672–9.

36. Provencher SW. Automatic quantitation of localized in vivo 1H spectra with LCModel. NMR Biomed 2001;14(4):260–4.

37. Doyle TJ, Pathak R, Wolinsky JS, et al. Automated proton spectroscopic image processing. J Magn Reson B 1995;106(1):58–63.

38. Maudsley AA, Wu Z, Meyerhoff DJ, et al. Automated processing for proton spectroscopic imaging using water reference deconvolution. Magn Reson Med 1994;31(6):589–95.

39. Mierisova S, Ala-Korpela M. MR spectroscopy quantitation: a review of frequency domain methods. NMR Biomed 2001;14(4):247–59.

40. Kaartinen J, Mierisova S, Oja JM, et al. Automated quantification of human brain metabolites by artificial neural network analysis from in vivo single-voxel 1H NMR spectra. J Magn Reson 1998; 134(1):176–9.

41. Hiltunen Y, Kaartinen J, Pulkkinen J, et al. Quantification of human brain metabolites from in vivo 1H NMR magnitude spectra using automated artificial neural network analysis. J Magn Reson 2002; 154(1):1–5.

42. Marshall I, Higinbotham J, Bruce S, et al. Use of Voigt lineshape for quantification of in vivo 1H spectra. Magn Reson Med 1997;37(5):651–7.

43. Bhat H, Sajja BR, Narayana PA. Fast quantification of proton magnetic resonance spectroscopic imaging with artificial neural networks. J Magn Reson 2006;183(1):110–22.

44. Naressi A, Couturier C, Devos JM, et al. Java-based graphical user interface for the MRUI quantitation package. MAGMA 2001;12(2–3):141–52.

45. Maudsley AA, Darkazanli A, Alger JR, et al. Comprehensive processing, display and analysis for in vivo MR spectroscopic imaging. NMR Biomed 2006;19(4):492–503.

46. Adams HP, Wagner S, Sobel DF, et al. Hypointense and hyperintense lesions on magnetic resonance imaging in secondary-progressive MS patients. Eur Neurol 1999;42(1):52–63.

47. Davie CA, Barker GJ, Thompson AJ, et al. 1H magnetic resonance spectroscopy of chronic cerebral white matter lesions and normal appearing white matter in multiple sclerosis. J Neurol Neurosurg Psychiatr 1997;63(6):736–42.

48. He J, Inglese M, Li BS, et al. Relapsing-remitting multiple sclerosis: metabolic abnormality in nonenhancing lesions and normal-appearing white matter at MR imaging: initial experience. Radiology 2005;234(1):211–7.

49. Arnold DL, De Stefano N, Narayanan S, et al. Proton MR spectroscopy in multiple sclerosis. Neuroimaging Clin N Am 2000;10(4):789–98, ix–x.

50. Wolinsky JS, Narayana PA, Fenstermacher MJ. Proton magnetic resonance spectroscopy in multiple sclerosis. Neurology 1990;40(11):1764–9.

51. Larsson HB, Christiansen P, Jensen M, et al. Localized in vivo proton spectroscopy in the brain of patients with multiple sclerosis. Magn Reson Med 1991;22(1):23–31.

52. Davie CA, Hawkins CP, Barker GJ, et al. Serial proton magnetic resonance spectroscopy in acute multiple sclerosis lesions. Brain 1994;117(Pt 1):49–58.

53. Trapp BD, Peterson J, Ransohoff RM, et al. Axonal transection in the lesions of multiple sclerosis. N Engl J Med 1998;338(5):278–85.

54. Reddy H, Narayanan S, Matthews PM, et al. Relating axonal injury to functional recovery in MS. Neurology 2000;54(1):236–9.

55. De Stefano N, Matthews PM, Arnold DL. Reversible decreases in N-acetylaspartate after acute brain injury. Magn Reson Med 1995;34(5):721–7.

56. Mader I, Roser W, Kappos L, et al. Serial proton MR spectroscopy of contrast-enhancing multiple sclerosis plaques: absolute metabolic values over 2 years during a clinical pharmacological study. AJNR Am J Neuroradiol 2000;21(7):1220–7.

57. Arnold DL, Matthews PM, Francis GS, et al. Proton magnetic resonance spectroscopic imaging for metabolic characterization of demyelinating plaques. Ann Neurol 1992;31(3):235–41.

58. De Stefano N, Matthews PM, Antel JP, et al. Chemical pathology of acute demyelinating lesions and its correlation with disability. Ann Neurol 1995;38(6):901–9.

59. Filippi M, Agosta F. Magnetization transfer MRI in multiple sclerosis. J Neuroimaging 2007;17(Suppl 1):22S–6S.

60. Rovaris M, Filippi M. Diffusion tensor MRI in multiple sclerosis. J Neuroimaging 2007;17(Suppl 1):27S–30S.

61. Fu L, Matthews PM, De Stefano N, et al. Imaging axonal damage of normal-appearing white matter in multiple sclerosis. Brain 1998;121(Pt 1):103–13.

62. Husted CA, Goodin DS, Hugg JW, et al. Biochemical alterations in multiple sclerosis lesions and normal-appearing white matter detected by in vivo 31P and 1H spectroscopic imaging. Ann Neurol 1994;36(2):157–65.

63. Narayanan S, Fu L, Pioro E, et al. Imaging of axonal damage in multiple sclerosis: spatial distribution of magnetic resonance imaging lesions. Ann Neurol 1997;41(3):385–91.

64. Sarchielli P, Presciutti O, Pelliccioli GP, et al. Absolute quantification of brain metabolites by proton magnetic resonance spectroscopy in normal-appearing white matter of multiple sclerosis patients. Brain 1999;122(Pt 3):513–21.

65. Bjartmar C, Kinkel RP, Kidd G, et al. Axonal loss in normal-appearing white matter in a patient with acute MS. Neurology 2001;57(7):1248–52.

66. Tartaglia MC, Narayanan S, De Stefano N, et al. Choline is increased in pre-lesional normal appearing white matter in multiple sclerosis. J Neurol 2002;249(10):1382–90.

67. Filippi M, Rocca MA, Martino G, et al. Magnetization transfer changes in the normal appearing white matter precede the appearance of enhancing lesions in patients with multiple sclerosis. Ann Neurol 1998;43(6):809–14.

68. Chard DT, Griffin CM, McLean MA, et al. Brain metabolite changes in cortical grey and normal-appearing white matter in clinically early relapsing-remitting multiple sclerosis. Brain 2002;125(Pt 10):2342–52.

69. Tiberio M, Chard DT, Altmann DR, et al. Metabolite changes in early relapsing-remitting multiple sclerosis. A two year follow-up study. J Neurol 2006;253(2):224–30.

70. Leary SM, Davie CA, Parker GJ, et al. 1H magnetic resonance spectroscopy of normal appearing white matter in primary progressive multiple sclerosis. J Neurol 1999;246(11):1023–6.

71. Inglese M, Li BS, Rusinek H, et al. Diffusely elevated cerebral choline and creatine in relapsing-remitting multiple sclerosis. Magn Reson Med 2003;50(1):190–5.

72. Suhy J, Rooney WD, Goodkin DE, et al. 1H MRSI comparison of white matter and lesions in primary progressive and relapsing-remitting MS. Mult Scler 2000;6(3):148–55.

73. Tourbah A, Stievenart JL, Abanou A, et al. Normal-appearing white matter in optic neuritis and multiple sclerosis: a comparative proton spectroscopy study. Neuroradiology 1999;41(10):738–43.

74. Fernando KT, McLean MA, Chard DT, et al. Elevated white matter myo-inositol in clinically isolated syndromes suggestive of multiple sclerosis. Brain 2004;127(Pt 6):1361–9.

75. Wattjes MP, Harzheim M, Lutterbey GG, et al. Axonal damage but no increased glial cell activity in the normal-appearing white matter of patients with clinically isolated syndromes suggestive of multiple

sclerosis using high-field magnetic resonance spectroscopy. AJNR Am J Neuroradiol 2007; 28(8):1517–22.

76. Wattjes MP, Harzheim M, Lutterbey GG, et al. High field MR imaging and 1H-MR spectroscopy in clinically isolated syndromes suggestive of multiple sclerosis: correlation between metabolic alterations and diagnostic MR imaging criteria. J Neurol 2008; 255(1):56–63.

77. Minagar A. Gray matter involvement in multiple sclerosis: a new window into pathogenesis. J Neuroimaging 2003;13(4):291–2.

78. Stadelmann C, Albert M, Wegner C, et al. Cortical pathology in multiple sclerosis. Curr Opin Neurol 2008;21(3):229–34.

79. Bedell BJ, Narayana PA. Implementation and evaluation of a new pulse sequence for rapid acquisition of double inversion recovery images for simultaneous suppression of white matter and CSF. J Magn Reson Imaging 1998;8(3):544–7.

80. Geurts JJ, Pouwels PJ, Uitdehaag BM, et al. Intracortical lesions in multiple sclerosis: improved detection with 3D double inversion-recovery MR imaging. Radiology 2005;236(1):254–60.

81. Geurts JJ, Bo L, Pouwels PJ, et al. Cortical lesions in multiple sclerosis: combined postmortem MR imaging and histopathology. AJNR Am J Neuroradiol 2005;26(3):572–7.

82. Nelson F, Poonawalla AH, Hou P, et al. Improved identification of intracortical lesions in multiple sclerosis with phase-sensitive inversion recovery in combination with fast double inversion recovery MR imaging. AJNR Am J Neuroradiol 2007;28(9): 1645–9.

83. Dehmeshki J, Chard DT, Leary SM, et al. The normal appearing grey matter in primary progressive multiple sclerosis: a magnetisation transfer imaging study. J Neurol 2003;250(1):67–74.

84. Rovaris M, Bozzali M, Iannucci G, et al. Assessment of normal-appearing white and gray matter in patients with primary progressive multiple sclerosis: a diffusion-tensor magnetic resonance imaging study. Arch Neurol 2002;59(9):1406–12.

85. Poonawalla AH, Hasan KM, Gupta RK, et al. Diffusion-tensor MR imaging of cortical lesions in multiple sclerosis: initial findings. Radiology 2008; 246(3):880–6.

86. Kapeller P, McLean MA, Griffin CM, et al. Preliminary evidence for neuronal damage in cortical grey matter and normal appearing white matter in short duration relapsing-remitting multiple sclerosis: a quantitative MR spectroscopic imaging study. J Neurol 2001;248(2):131–8.

87. Sijens PE, Mostert JP, Oudkerk M, et al. (1)H MR spectroscopy of the brain in multiple sclerosis subtypes with analysis of the metabolite concentrations

in gray and white matter: initial findings. Eur Radiol 2006;16(2):489–95.

88. Van Au Duong M, Audoin B, Le Fur Y, et al. Relationships between gray matter metabolic abnormalities and white matter inflammation in patients at the very early stage of MS: a MRSI study. J Neurol 2007;254(7):914–23.

89. Geurts JJ, Reuling IE, Vrenken H, et al. MR spectroscopic evidence for thalamic and hippocampal, but not cortical, damage in multiple sclerosis. Magn Reson Med 2006;55(3):478–83.

90. Adalsteinsson E, Langer-Gould A, Homer RJ, et al. Gray matter N-acetyl aspartate deficits in secondary progressive but not relapsing-remitting multiple sclerosis. AJNR Am J Neuroradiol 2003;24(10): 1941–5.

91. Sarchielli P, Presciutti O, Tarducci R, et al. Localized (1)H magnetic resonance spectroscopy in mainly cortical gray matter of patients with multiple sclerosis. J Neurol 2002;249(7):902–10.

92. Cifelli A, Arridge M, Jezzard P, et al. Thalamic neurodegeneration in multiple sclerosis. Ann Neurol 2002;52(5):650–3.

93. Bakshi R, Benedict RH, Bermel RA, et al. T2 hypointensity in the deep gray matter of patients with multiple sclerosis: a quantitative magnetic resonance imaging study. Arch Neurol 2002;59(1): 62–8.

94. Wylezinska M, Cifelli A, Jezzard P, et al. Thalamic neurodegeneration in relapsing-remitting multiple sclerosis. Neurology 2003;60(12):1949–54.

95. Birnbaum G, Leist TP, Lublin FD. Commentary I: pathophysiologic construct for neuronal degeneration/regeneration in multiple sclerosis. Neurology 2007;68(Suppl 3):S2–4.

96. Gonen O, Catalaa I, Babb JS, et al. Total brain N-acetylaspartate: a new measure of disease load in MS. Neurology 2000;54(1):15–9.

97. Rovaris M, Gallo A, Falini A, et al. Axonal injury and overall tissue loss are not related in primary progressive multiple sclerosis. Arch Neurol 2005; 62(6):898–902.

98. Ge Y, Gonen O, Inglese M, et al. Neuronal cell injury precedes brain atrophy in multiple sclerosis. Neurology 2004;62(4):624–7.

99. Filippi M, Bozzali M, Rovaris M, et al. Evidence for widespread axonal damage at the earliest clinical stage of multiple sclerosis. Brain 2003;126(Pt 2): 433–7.

100. Tartaglino LM, Friedman DP, Flanders AE, et al. Multiple sclerosis in the spinal cord: MR appearance and correlation with clinical parameters. Radiology 1995;195(3):725–32.

101. Bastianello S, Paolillo A, Giugni E, et al. MRI of spinal cord in MS. J Neurovirol 2000;6(Suppl 2): S130–3.

102. Ganter P, Prince C, Esiri MM. Spinal cord axonal loss in multiple sclerosis: a post-mortem study. Neuropathol Appl Neurobiol 1999;25(6):459–67.

103. DeLuca GC, Ebers GC, Esiri MM. Axonal loss in multiple sclerosis: a pathological survey of the corticospinal and sensory tracts. Brain 2004;127(Pt 5): 1009–18.

104. Blamire AM, Cader S, Lee M, et al. Axonal damage in the spinal cord of multiple sclerosis patients detected by magnetic resonance spectroscopy. Magn Reson Med 2007;58(5):880–5.

105. Marliani AF, Clementi V, Albini-Riccioli L, et al. Quantitative proton magnetic resonance spectroscopy of the human cervical spinal cord at 3 Tesla. Magn Reson Med 2007;57(1):160–3.

106. Kendi AT, Tan FU, Kendi M, et al. MR spectroscopy of cervical spinal cord in patients with multiple sclerosis. Neuroradiology 2004;46(9):764–9.

107. Ciccarelli O, Wheeler-Kingshott CA, McLean MA, et al. Spinal cord spectroscopy and diffusion-based tractography to assess acute disability in multiple sclerosis. Brain 2007;130(Pt 8):2220–31.

108. Arnold DL. Evidence for neuroprotection and remyelination using imaging techniques. Neurology 2007;68(22 Suppl 3):S83–90 [discussion: S86–91].

109. Khan O, Shen Y, Caon C, et al. Axonal metabolic recovery and potential neuroprotective effect of glatiramer acetate in relapsing-remitting multiple sclerosis. Mult Scler 2005;11(6):646–51.

110. Comi G, Filippi M, Wolinsky JS. European/Canadian multicenter, double-blind, randomized, placebo-controlled study of the effects of glatiramer acetate on magnetic resonance imaging–measured disease activity and burden in patients with relapsing multiple sclerosis. European/Canadian glatiramer acetate study group. Ann Neurol 2001; 49(3):290–7.

111. Paty DW, Li DK. Interferon beta-1b is effective in relapsing-remitting multiple sclerosis. II. MRI analysis results of a multicenter, randomized, double-blind, placebo-controlled trial. UBC MS/MRI study group and the IFNB multiple sclerosis study group. Neurology 1993;43(4):662–7.

112. Narayanan S, Caramanos Z, Arnold D. The effect of glatiramer acetate treatment on axonal integrity in multiple sclerosis [abstract]. Mult Scler 2004; 10(Suppl 2):S256, Abstract P633.

113. Khan O, Shen Y, Bao F, et al. Long-term study of brain ^{1}H-MRS study in multiple sclerosis: effect of glatiramer acetate therapy on axonal metabolic function and feasibility of long-term H-MRS monitoring in multiple sclerosis. J Neuroimaging 2008; 18(3):314–9.

114. Sajja BR, Narayana PA, Wolinsky JS, et al. Longitudinal magnetic resonance spectroscopic imaging of primary progressive multiple sclerosis patients treated with glatiramer acetate: multicenter study. Mult Scler 2008;14(1):73–80.

115. Wolinsky JS, Narayana PA, O'Connor P, et al. Glatiramer acetate in primary progressive multiple sclerosis: results of a multinational, multicenter, double-blind, placebo-controlled trial. Ann Neurol 2007;61(1):14–24.

116. Schubert F, Seifert F, Elster C, et al. Serial 1H-MRS in relapsing-remitting multiple sclerosis: effects of interferon-beta therapy on absolute metabolite concentrations. MAGMA 2002;14(3):213–22.

117. Sarchielli P, Presciutti O, Tarducci R, et al. 1H-MRS in patients with multiple sclerosis undergoing treatment with interferon beta-1a: results of a preliminary study. J Neurol Neurosurg Psychiatr 1998;64(2):204–12.

118. Narayanan S, De Stefano N, Francis GS, et al. Axonal metabolic recovery in multiple sclerosis patients treated with interferon beta-1b. J Neurol 2001;248(11):979–86.

Functional MR Imaging in Multiple Sclerosis

Massimo Filippi, MD*, M.A. Rocca, MD

KEYWORDS

- Multiple sclerosis • Functional magnetic resonance imaging
- Adaptation • Motor system • Visual system • Cognition

Over the past decade, conventional and modern structural MR imaging techniques have been extensively used to study patients who have multiple sclerosis (MS) with the ultimate goal of increasing the understanding of the mechanisms responsible for the accumulation of irreversible disability.[1,2] In summary, the application of MR imaging techniques to the definition of MS pathophysiology has shown that: (1) MS-related damage is not restricted to T2-visible lesions, but it involves diffusely the normal-appearing white matter (NAWM) and gray matter (GM); (2) the neurodegenerative component of the disease is not a late phenomenon and it is not fully driven by inflammatory demyelination; and (3) axonal damage contributes significantly to the clinical manifestations of the disease. Despite this, however, the magnitude of the correlation between MR imaging and clinical findings remains suboptimal.

Among the reasons for such a discrepancy, a variable intra- and intersubject effectiveness of reparative and recovery mechanisms following MS-related tissue injury is increasingly being considered. In this context, brain plasticity, a well-known feature of the human brain, which is likely to result from the interplay of several different substrates (such as increased axonal expression of sodium channels, synaptic rearrangement, increased recruitment of parallel existing pathways or "latent" connections, and reorganization of distant sites), is viewed as a major factor with an adaptive role in limiting the functional outcome of axonal loss in MS.

The signal changes seen during functional MR (fMR) imaging studies depend on the blood oxygen level–dependent (BOLD) mechanism, which, in turn, involves changes of the transverse magnetization relaxation time—either T2* in a gradient echo sequence, or T2 in spin echo sequence.[3] Local increases in neuronal activity result in an increase of blood flow and oxygen consumption. The increase of blood flow is greater than the oxygen consumption, thus determining an increased ratio between oxygenated and deoxygenated hemoglobin, which enhances the MR imaging signal.[3]

This article summarizes the main contributions to the understanding of MS pathobiology gained by the use of fMR imaging with different paradigms of stimulation.

GENERAL CONSIDERATIONS

The main problem in the interpretation of fMR imaging studies in diseased people is that the observed changes might be biased by disease-driven differences in task performance between patients and controls. Clearly, this is a major issue in MS, which typically causes impairment of various functional systems. Despite providing several important pieces of information, therefore, the value of the earliest fMR imaging studies of patients who have MS[4–10] has to be weighed against this background. For this reason, the most recent fMR imaging studies in MS have been based on larger and more selected patient groups than the seminal studies. These latter studies have investigated the brain patterns of cortical activations during the performance of several motor, visual, and cognitive tasks in patients who have all the major clinical phenotypes of the disease. One of the most solid conclusions that can be drawn from

Neuroimaging Research Unit, Department of Neurology, San Raffaele Scientific Institute and University, Via Olgettina, 60-20132, Milan, Italy
* Corresponding author.
E-mail address: filippi.massimo@hsr.it (M. Filippi).

Neuroimag Clin N Am 19 (2009) 59–70
doi:10.1016/j.nic.2008.08.004
1052-5149/08/$ – see front matter © 2008 Elsevier Inc. All rights reserved.

fMR imaging studies of MS is that cortical reorganization does occur in patients affected by this condition. The correlation between various measures of structural MS damage and the extent of cortical activations also suggests an adaptive role of such cortical changes in contributing to clinical recovery and maintaining a normal level of functioning in patients who have MS, despite the presence of axonal/neuronal loss, and, conversely, their failure or exhaustion with increasing disease duration or burden is likely to contribute to the accrual of irreversible disability.

THE VISUAL SYSTEM

The method usually applied to investigate the visual system in MS and related disorders consists of the application of an 8 Hz photic stimulation to one or both eyes.[5,9–15]

Acute Optic Neuritis Suggestive of Multiple Sclerosis

Compared with healthy controls, patients who have recovered from a single episode of acute unilateral optic neuritis, when the clinically affected eye is studied, show an extensive activation of the visual network, including the claustrum, lateral temporal and posterior parietal cortices, and thalamus, in addition to the primary visual cortex.[9] When the unaffected eye is stimulated, only activations of the visual cortex and the right insula/claustrum are observed.[9] In addition, the volume of the extra-occipital activation is strongly correlated with the latency of the visual evoked potential (VEP) P100, suggesting that the functional reorganization of the cortex might represent an adaptive response to a persistently abnormal visual input.[9]

Subsequent studies[11,12,14] have confirmed the results of this seminal report. Toosy and colleagues[11] used a longer photic stimulation epoch to better elucidate the nature of the abnormal extra-occipital response, which had a peak during the OFF phase of the stimulation paradigm. The results of this study confirm the original finding of a phase-dependent increase of the BOLD signal in the extra-occipital regions during the baseline condition. Russ and colleagues[12] used fMR imaging and VEP to monitor the functional recovery after an acute unilateral optic neuritis and found a strong relationship between fMR imaging and VEP latencies, suggesting that fMR imaging can contribute to the assessment of the temporal evolution of the visual deficits during recovery, either natural or modified by treatment. Levin and colleagues[14] showed reduced activation of the primary visual cortex and increased activation of the lateral occipital complex (LOC) in eight

subjects who recovered clinically from an episode of optic neuritis, but who still had prolonged VEP latencies in comparison with healthy controls. More recently, in a 1-year follow up study, Toosy and colleagues,[11] using a novel technique that modeled the fMR imaging response and optic nerve structure together with clinical function, demonstrated a potential adaptive role of cortical reorganization within the extrastriate visual areas, which are regions involved in higher-order visual processing, early after optic neuritis. In addition, at 3 months more severe optic nerve damage was associated with an increased fMR imaging response in the bilateral temporal cortices, whereas at 1 year, the right temporal cortex correlation reversed.[11] These results illustrate how the same regions may play different roles at different times during recovery, reflecting the complexity of brain plasticity and the demyelinating process. This notion has been supported by a recent region-of-interest longitudinal study[15] that demonstrated dynamic changes of the fMR imaging response following visual stimulation not only in V1, V2, and the LOC, but also in the lateral geniculate nucleus (LGN) in patients who had isolate acute optic neuritis (**Fig. 1**).

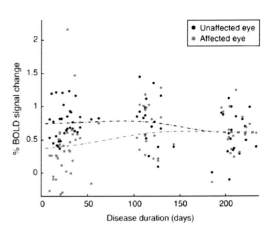

Fig. 1. Mean LGN activation during stimulation of the affected and unaffected eye over time. The dash-dotted lines indicate weighted moving averages for the affected eye (*red*) and unaffected eye (*black*). During recovery there is a significant increase in LGN BOLD signal from stimulation of the affected eye. The LGN BOLD signal from stimulation of the unaffected eye decreases over time in a stepwise fashion. Post hoc analysis showed this decrease to be significant. The BOLD signal changes for the affected and unaffected eye level off at a similar positive value as time increases (*From* Korsholm K, Madsen KH, Frederiksen JL, et al. Recovery from optic neuritis: an ROI-based analysis of LGN and visual cortical areas. Brain 2007;130:1248; with permission.)

Relapsing-Remitting Multiple Sclerosis

In patients who had established MS and a relapsing-remitting (RR) course with a unilateral optic neuritis, a reduced recruitment of the visual cortex after stimulation of the affected and the unaffected eyes was found when compared with healthy subjects. On average, patients who had complete clinical recovery showed a greater visual cortex recruitment than those who had poor or no recovery, although the extent of the activation remained reduced compared with that of controls.[5] A more recent study[10] of nine patients who had a previous optic neuritis showed that these patients not only have a reduced activation of the V1, but also a reduced fMR imaging percentage signal change in this region, again suggesting an abnormality of the synaptic input.

MOTOR SYSTEM

The investigation of the motor system in patients who have MS has mainly focused on the analysis of the performance of simple motor tasks with the dominant right upper limbs.[6–8,16–35] Such tasks were either self-paced or paced by a metronome. A few studies assessed the performance of simple motor tasks with the dominant right lower limbs,[19,22,28] and even fewer studies have investigated the performance of more complex tasks, including phasic movements of dominant hand and foot,[22,36] object manipulation,[37] and visuomotor integration tasks.[38]

Clinically Isolated Syndromes Suggestive of Multiple Sclerosis

An altered brain pattern of movement-associated cortical activations, characterized by an increased recruitment of the contralateral primary sensorimotor cortex (SMC) during the performance of simple tasks[18,22] and by the recruitment of additional classic and higher-order sensorimotor areas during the performance of more complex tasks[22] has been demonstrated in patients who have clinically isolated syndromes (CIS) suggestive of MS. The clinical and conventional MR imaging follow-up of these patients has shown that, at disease onset, patients who have CIS with a subsequent evolution to clinically definite MS tend to recruit a more widespread sensorimotor network than those who do not have short-term disease evolution.[23] These findings support the notion that, although increased recruitment of a widespread sensorimotor network contributes to limiting the impact of structural damage during the course of MS, its early activation might be counterproductive, because it might result in an early exhaustion of the adaptive properties of the brain.

Relapsing-Remitting Multiple Sclerosis

An increased recruitment of several sensorimotor areas, mainly located in the cerebral hemisphere ipsilateral to the limb that performs the task, has been demonstrated in patients who have early RRMS and a previous episode of hemiparesis.[24] In patients who had similar characteristics, but who presented with an episode of optic neuritis, this increased recruitment involved sensorimotor areas that were mainly located in the contralateral cerebral hemisphere.[25]

In patients who have RRMS, functional cortical changes, mainly characterized by an increased recruitment of classic motor areas, including the primary SMC, the supplementary motor area (SMA), and the secondary sensorimotor cortex (SII), have been shown during the performance of simple motor[6–8,17] and visuomotor integration tasks.[38] More recently, abnormal functional connectivity of the motor network has also been demonstrated to occur in these patients.[30,35]

Progressive Multiple Sclerosis

Movement-associated cortical changes, characterized by the activation of highly specialized cortical areas, have been described in patients who have secondary progressive (SP) MS[19] during the performance of a simple motor task and in patients who have primary progressive (PP) MS during the performance of active[16,28] and passive[36] motor experiments.

COGNITION

Recent fMR imaging studies have suggested that functional cortical changes might have an adaptive role also in limiting MS-related cognitive impairment.[39–55] Several cognitive domains have been investigated in patients who have MS with fMR imaging. Working memory has been the most extensively studied by using the Paced Auditory Serial Addition Test (PASAT) or the Paced Visual Serial Addition Task (PVSAT)[39–42,47,51] (which also involves sustained attention, information processing speed, and simple calculation), the n-back task,[46,48–50,52] or a task adapted from the Sternberg paradigm.[44] Additional cognitive domains including attention[45] and planning[55] have also been interrogated.

Clinically Isolated Syndromes Suggestive of Multiple Sclerosis

In patients who have CIS, an altered pattern of cortical activations has been described during the performance of the PASAT,[42,43] confirming the presence of cortical reorganization at the earliest clinical stage of the disease.

Relapsing-Remitting Multiple Sclerosis

During the performance of the PVSAT, patients who have RRMS with a preserved task performance have increased activations of several regions located in the frontal and parietal lobes, bilaterally.[39] Similarly, cognitively preserved RRMS showed, during an n-back test, a reduced activation of the core areas of the working memory circuitry (including prefrontal and parietal regions) and an increased recruitment of other regions within and beyond the typical working memory circuitry (including areas in the frontal, parietal, temporal and occipital lobes).[50] An increased recruitment of several cortical areas (in particular in the frontal and temporal lobes) has also been shown in patients who have RRMS and mild clinical disability during the performance of a simple cognitive task,[47] and when testing rehearsal within working memory.[44] In this latter case, the degree of right hemisphere recruitment was strongly related to the neuropsychologic performance.[44] Other studies,[48,49,53] which also investigated working memory, demonstrated that compared with controls, patients who have MS have (1) an increased recruitment of regions related to sensorimotor functions and anterior attentional/executive components of the working memory system, and (2) a reduced activation of several regions in the right cerebellar hemisphere.[53]

A recent fMR imaging study[52] applied an analysis of functional connectivity to investigate n-back functional correlates in a group of 21 patients who had RRMS. Compared with controls, patients had relatively reduced activations of the superior frontal and anterior cingulate gyri, and a smaller increase of activation with greater task complexity. This finding suggests a reduced functional reserve for cognition relevant to memory in these patients. In addition, the analysis of functional connectivity revealed increased correlations between right dorsolateral prefrontal and superior frontal/anterior cingulate activations in controls, and increased correlations between activations of the right and left prefrontal cortices in patients. This finding suggests that an altered interhemispheric interaction between dorsal and lateral prefrontal regions may yet be an additional adaptive mechanism distinct from recruitment of novel processing regions.[52]

Benign Multiple Sclerosis

Using a 3.0 T scanner, more significant activations of several areas of the cognitive network involved in the performance of the Stroop test have been demonstrated in cognitively preserved patients who have benign MS (BMS) (**Fig. 2**).[54] Patients who had BMS also showed an increased connectivity between several cortical areas of the cognitive network (including the left and right inferior frontal gyri [IFG], the anterior cingulate cortex, and the left SII), and between some of these areas and the right cerebellum, and a decreased connectivity between some other areas (including the left SII, the prefrontal cortex, and the right cerebellum) and the anterior cingulate cortex. These results suggest an altered interhemispheric balance in favor of the right hemisphere in patients who have BMS in comparison with healthy controls, when performing cognitive tasks.

FUNCTIONAL MR IMAGING CHANGES OF THE SPINAL CORD

Although BOLD fMR imaging of the spinal cord has provided reliable results in healthy subjects,[56] several studies[56] suggested that the exploitation of the so-called "signal enhancement by extravascular protons" (SEEP) effect rather than the classic BOLD effect might be more suitable for the assessment of spinal cord activity. Such an effect is proposed to arise from a local modification in fluid balance that may result from changes in perfusion pressure, production of extracellular fluid, cellular swelling, and maintenance of ion and neurotransmitter concentrations at sites of neuronal activity.[56] Following a tactile stimulation of the palm of the right hand, significant task-related signal change in the ipsilateral cervical cord (especially at C6 and C7) has been detected in 12 right-handed healthy subjects.[57]

Two studies have interrogated cervical cord neuronal activity during a proprioceptive[58] and a tactile[59] stimulation of the right upper limb in patients who have relapsing MS. In the first study,[58] in comparison with controls, patients who had MS had an higher average fMR imaging signal change of the overall cord and of the anterior section of the right cord at C5 and left cord at C5-C6. In the second study, compared with controls, patients who had MS showed a 20% higher cord fMR imaging signal change (**Fig. 3**)[59] and a different topographic distribution of fMR imaging changes at the level of the different portions of the cervical cord (mainly characterized by an

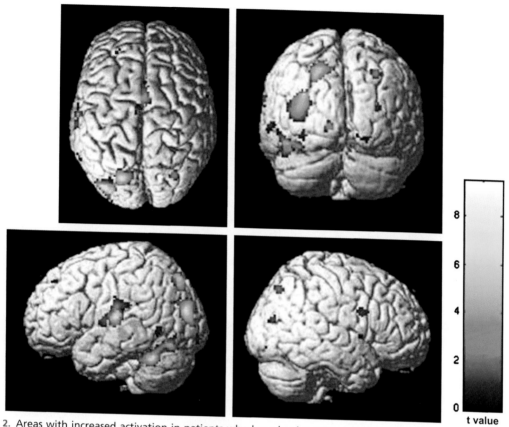

Fig. 2. Areas with increased activation in patients who have benign MS compared with healthy controls during the Stroop interference condition (random effect interaction analysis, ANOVA, $P<.05$ corrected for multiple comparisons). Note that the color-coded activations have been superimposed on a rendered brain and normalized into standard statistical parametric mapping space (neurologic convention) (*From* Rocca MA, Valsasina P, Ceccarelli A, et al. Structural and functional MRI correlates of Stroop control in benign MS. Hum Brain Mapp 2007 Nov 27 [Epub ahead of print]; with permission.)

activation of regions located in the anterior and the left portions). Such an over-recruitment of the ipsilateral posterior cervical cord associated to a reduced functional lateralization suggests an abnormal function of the spinal relay interneurons in patients who have MS.

CORRELATIONS BETWEEN THE EXTENT OF FUNCTIONAL CORTICAL REORGANIZATION AND STRUCTURAL MR DAMAGE IN MULTIPLE SCLEROSIS

Most of the studies reviewed in the previous paragraphs found a relationship between the extent of

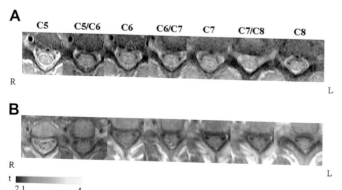

Fig. 3. Illustrative activation maps (color coded for *t* values) of cervical cord on axial proton density-weighted spin-echo images from C5 to C8, from a healthy control (*A*) and a patient who has MS (*B*) during a tactile stimulation of the right palm of hand. R, right; L, left.

fMR imaging activations and measures of tissue damage.[6–8,16–20,25,28,38,40,43,45,47]

An increased recruitment of several brain regions with increasing T2 lesion load has been shown in patients who have RRMS[6–8,40,47] and PPMS.[28] The severity of intrinsic T2-visible lesion damage, measured using T1-weighted images,[25] magnetization transfer (MT), and diffusion tensor (DT) MR imaging,[17] has been found to modulate the activity of some cortical areas in these patients. The severity of normal-appearing brain tissue injury, measured using proton MR spectroscopy,[7,8,18] MT MR imaging,[16,17,40,43] and DT MR imaging,[16,18,20] is another factor found to be associated with an increased recruitment of motor- and cognitive-related brain regions, as shown by studies of patients at presentation who had CIS suggestive of MS,[18,40,43] patients who had RRMS and variable degrees of clinical disability,[7,8,17,20] patients who had PPMS,[16] and patients who had SPMS.[7,8] Finally, subtle GM damage, which goes undetected when using conventional MR imaging, may also influence functional cortical recruitment, as demonstrated for the motor system in patients who had RRMS[38] or SPMS[19] and in patients who had clinically definite MS and nonspecific (fewer than three focal WM lesions) conventional MR imaging findings.[20] In patients who have MS who are cognitively intact, the increased activation of a left prefrontal region during the counting Stroop task has been correlated with the normalized brain parenchymal volume.[45]

Structural damage of WM pathways that connect functionally relevant areas for a given task has been shown to modify the observed brain patterns of cortical activations in patients who have MS. Damage to the corticospinal tract[25,26] and damage to the corpus callosum (**Fig. 4**)[27,30,60,61] have been related to a more bilateral movement-associated brain pattern of cortical activations.

The recent development of diffusion-based tractography methods that allow the pathways connecting different central nervous system (CNS) structures and their application to patients who have MS to be defined with precision resulted in an improvement of the correlation between structural and functional abnormalities. Recent work has combined measures of abnormal functional connectivity with DT MR measures of damage within selected WM fiber bundles in patients who had RRMS[35] and BMS.[54] In patients who had RRMS and no clinical disability,[35] measures of abnormal functional connectivity of the motor network were correlated with structural MR imaging metrics of tissue damage of the corticospinal and the dentatorubrothalamic tracts, whereas no correlation was found with measures of damage

to "not-motor" WM fiber bundles. In patients who had BMS,[54] measures of abnormal functional connectivity of the cognitive network were moderately correlated with structural MR imaging metrics of tissue damage within intra- and interhemispheric cognitive-related WM fiber bundles, whereas no correlation was found with the extent of injury to the other fiber bundles studied. These results suggest that functional cortical changes in patients who have BMS might represent an adaptive response driven by damage to critical WM structures.

In patients who have PPMS[16] a relationship has been demonstrated between the severity of spinal cord pathology, measured using MT MR imaging, and the extent of movement-associated cortical activations. In relapsing patients who have MS, average signal change of the entire cervical cord was found to be correlated with the extent of cord and brain tissue damage.[58]

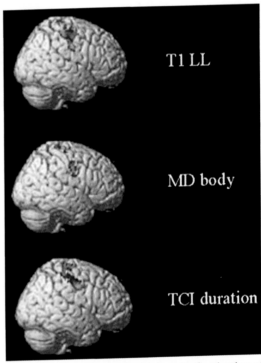

Fig. 4. Correlation between the extent of activation of the ipsilateral primary motor cortex (iM1) and damage of the corpus callosum (CC) in patients who have RRMS. Three predictors were found to be significantly correlated (cluster-level corrected *P*<.05): mean diffusivity (MD) in the body of CC (directly), T1 lesion load (LL) (directly), and transcallosal inhibition (TCI) duration (inversely) (*From* Lenzi D, Conte A, Mainero C, et al. Effect of corpus callosum damage on ipsilateral motor activation in patients with multiple sclerosis: a functional and anatomical study. Hum Brain Mapp 2007;28:641; with permission.)

ROLE OF FUNCTIONAL CORTICAL REORGANIZATION IN MULTIPLE SCLEROSIS

Although the actual role of cortical reorganization on the clinical manifestations of MS remains to be established, the correlation found between fMR imaging measures of abnormal activations and quantitative MR imaging metrics of structural brain and cord injury suggests that, at least in some phases of the disease, an increased recruitment of the cortical network might contribute in limiting the functional impact of MS-related damage.

The notion that an increased recruitment of areas that are usually activated by healthy individuals when performing different/more complex tasks might be one of the mechanisms playing a role in MS recovery/maintenance of motor function has been highlighted by the results of two recent experiments.[34,37] The first showed that patients who have MS, during the performance of a simple motor task, activate some regions that are part of a fronto-parietal circuit, whose recruitment occurs typically in healthy subjects during object manipulation.[34] The second demonstrated activations of regions that are part of the mirror-neuron system in patients who have MS during the performance of the same task.[37]

An fMR imaging study of patients who had different disease phenotypes showed that movement-associated cortical reorganization varies across patients at different stages of the disease,[31] suggesting that the adaptive role of brain plasticity in limiting the clinical consequences of widespread disease-related tissue damage might change with disease progression. In particular, this study demonstrated that more areas typically devoted to motor tasks are recruited in the early phase of MS, then a bilateral activation of these regions is seen, and later in the disease course areas that healthy people recruit to perform novel or complex tasks are activated, perhaps in an attempt to limit the functional consequences of accumulating tissue damage.

Several studies suggested that an increased cortical recruitment might not always be beneficial for patients who have MS. In patients who have PPMS, it has been suggested that the lack or exhaustion of the classic adaptive mechanisms might be among the factors responsible for an unfavorable clinical evolution.[16,28,36] Similar findings have led to identical conclusions in patients who had cognitive decline,[46] in whom a reallocation of neuronal resources and the inefficiency of neuronal processes have been associated with the extent of structural tissue damage.

Finally, the comparison of the movement-associated brain patterns of cortical activations between RRMS patients complaining of reversible fatigue after interferon (IFN)β-1a administration and those who did not have such a symptom demonstrated an association between the presence of fatigue and an increased recruitment of several areas of the motor network, including the thalamus, the cingulum, and several regions located in the frontal lobes, such as the SMA and the primary SMC, bilaterally (**Fig. 5**).[32] These results suggest that the over-recruitment of brain networks in MS might, at least to some degree, have a detrimental effect.

USE OF FMR IMAGING TO ASSESS LONGITUDINAL CHANGES OF CORTICAL REORGANIZATION

Dynamic functional changes have been described in a patient who had MS after an acute relapse.[7] These results have been confirmed and extended by a recent study that assessed the early cortical changes following acute motor relapses secondary to pseudotumoral lesions in 12 patients who had MS and the evolution over time of cortical reorganization in a subgroup of these patients.[33] In this study,[33] short-term cortical changes were mainly characterized by the recruitment of pathways in the unaffected hemisphere. A recovery of function of the primary SMC of the affected hemisphere was found in patients who had clinical improvement, whereas in patients who did not have clinical recovery there was a persistent recruitment of the primary SMC of the unaffected hemisphere. This finding suggests that the restoration of function of motor areas of the affected hemisphere might be a critical factor for a favorable clinical outcome.

A longitudinal (time interval of 15–26 months) fMR imaging study of the motor system has been conducted in a group of patients who had early RRMS.[62] Patients exhibited greater bilateral activations than controls in both fMR imaging studies. Although no significant difference between the two fMR imaging scans was observed in controls, a reduction of the functional activity of the ipsilateral SMC and the contralateral cerebellum was seen in patients at follow-up. Moreover, activation changes in ipsilateral motor areas correlated inversely with age, extent, and progression of T1 lesion load, and occurrence of a new relapse, suggesting that younger patients with less structural brain damage and a favorable clinical course demonstrate brain plasticity that follows a more lateralized pattern of brain activations.[62]

Only a few fMR imaging studies have been performed to monitor the effect of treatment in

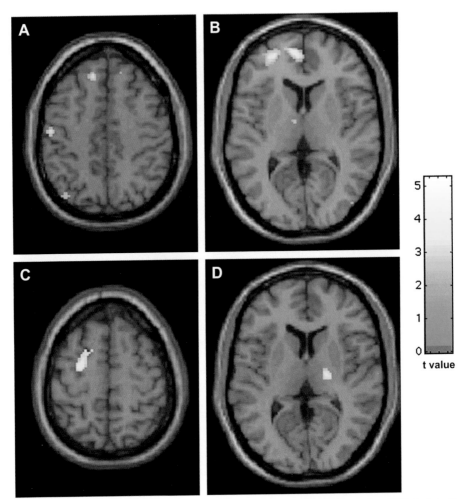

Fig. 5. Relative cortical activations of patients who had MS with reversible fatigue after IFNβ-1a injection during the performance of a simple motor task with their clinically unimpaired and fully normal functioning, dominant right hands. At entry (A, B) (when they did not complain of fatigue), compared with patients who had MS without reversible fatigue, these patients showed an increased recruitment of the contralateral primary SMC (A), the thalamus (B), the superior frontal sulcus (A, B), and the cingulate motor area (B). At day 1 (C, D) (after IFNβ-1a administration, when fatigue was present), compared with patients who had MS without fatigue, these patients showed increased recruitment of the ipsilateral thalamus (D), and contralateral middle frontal gyrus (C). Note that the color-coded activations have been superimposed on a high-resolution T1-weighted scan obtained from a single, healthy subject and normalized into standard statistical parametric mapping space (neurologic convention) (From Rocca MA, Agosta F, Colombo B, et al. fMRI changes in relapsing-remitting multiple sclerosis patients complaining of fatigue after IFNβ-1a injection. Hum Brain Mapp 2007;28:379; with permission.)

MS.[45,63,64] A preliminary study of five patients tested the effect of acute administration of rivastigmine, a central cholinesterase inhibitor, on the pattern of brain activations during the performance of a cognitive task (Stroop task).[45] After treatment administration, a relative normalization of the abnormal Stroop-associated brain activations was observed in patients, whereas no change in the pattern of brain activations was seen in any of the four healthy controls studied. In patients who had MS, increased activation of the ipsilateral primary SMC and SMA has also been observed after the administration of a single dose of 3,4-diaminopyridine (a potassium channel blocker), suggesting that this treatment may modulate brain motor activity in patients who have MS, probably by enhancing excitatory synaptic transmission.[63] A recent study analyzed how the motor network responds to training in patients who have MS with mild motor impairment of the right upper extremity.[64] Before training, patients who had MS had a more prominent activation of the contralateral dorsal premotor cortex during thumb movements when compared with controls. After training, unlike the control group, patients who had MS did not exhibit task-specific reductions in the activation of the contralateral primary SMC and adjacent parietal association cortices. The absence of training-dependent reductions in activations supports the notion that patients who have MS have a decreased capacity to optimize recruitment of the motor network with practice.

FMR IMAGING IN MULTICENTER STUDIES

Recently, the potential of fMR imaging in prospective multicenter studies has been interrogated in an international collaborative study.[65] To this aim, 56 patients who have MS and 60 age-matched, healthy controls have been recruited and studied at eight sites during the performance of a simple motor task. Compared with controls, patients who had MS had more significant activations bilaterally in brain regions including the pre- and postcentral, inferior and superior frontal, cingulate and superior temporal gyri and insula. Both patients and healthy controls showed greater brain activations of the ipsilateral precentral and IFG with increasing age. In addition, patients also showed a greater brain recruitment of the anterior cingulate gyrus and the bilateral ventral striatum with less hand dexterity. This large fMR imaging study over a broadly selected MS patient population confirms that movement demands significantly greater cognitive resource allocation in patients who have MS than in healthy people and suggests an age-related difference in brain response to the disease. These observations add to the evidence that brain functional responses contribute to the modulation of clinical expression of MS pathology and demonstrate the feasibility of multisite fMR imaging studies in MS. More recently, abnormalities of effective connectivity in the same subjects have been described.[66] This analysis demonstrated enhanced cortico-cortical shorter-range connectivities and impairment of long-distance connectivities in patients who had MS in comparison with healthy controls,[66] and showed that large multicenter fMR imaging studies of effective connectivity changes in diseased people are feasible, thus facilitating studies with sample size large enough for robust outcomes. Clearly, these findings set the stage for large-scale trials of neurorehabilitation and neuroprotection in MS.

UNRESOLVED ISSUES AND FUTURE PERSPECTIVES

fMR imaging is not without limitations. First, despite a relatively high spatial resolution, its temporal resolution is still lower than that of physiologic changes that are actually occurring in the CNS. Second, it is time consuming, in particular when obtained in combination with other sequences, and its acquisition needs to be standardized. Third, caution must be exercised when interpreting fMR imaging results obtained from pathology because various factors, including abnormalities of the BOLD effect related to inflammatory lesions, could affect the reliability of the data across sessions. Finally, conclusions are usually driven from the analysis of a single task in selected groups of individuals and, as a consequence, may not be generalized to the overall patient population.

The development of fMR imaging paradigms capable of providing useful information in disabled patients might increase the role of this technique in the assessment of MS pathobiology. In addition, because preliminary results indicate the feasibility of fMR imaging of the spinal cord, it is hoped that this technique will be successfully applied to the study of patients who have MS with different degrees of disability. Finally, additional longitudinal fMR imaging studies are warranted to define the temporal evolution of functional cortical changes in the different MS phenotypes, and their role in limiting the clinical consequences of increasing tissue damage. Such longitudinal fMR imaging studies would also enable us to monitor the effect of motor and cognitive rehabilitation and that of pharmacologic therapies in enhancing any beneficial effect of natural adaptive plasticity of the human CNS.

REFERENCES

1. Filippi M, Rocca MA. Magnetization transfer magnetic resonance imaging in the assessment of neurological diseases. J Neuroimaging 2004;14: 303–13 [Review].
2. Filippi M, Rocca MA, Comi G. The use of quantitative magnetic-resonance-based techniques to monitor the evolution of multiple sclerosis. Lancet Neurol 2003;2:337–46.
3. Ogawa S, Menon RS, Tank DW, et al. Functional brain mapping by blood oxygenation level-dependent contrast magnetic resonance imaging. A comparison of signal characteristics with a biophysical model. Biophys J 1993;64:803–12.
4. Clanet M, Berry I, Boulanouar K. Functional imaging in multiple sclerosis. Int Mult Scler J 1997;4:26–32.
5. Rombouts SA, Lazeron RH, Scheltens P, et al. Visual activation patterns in patients with optic neuritis: an fMRI pilot study. Neurology 1998;50:1896–9.
6. Lee MA, Reddy H, Johansen-Berg H, et al. The motor cortex shows adaptive functional changes to brain injury from multiple sclerosis. Ann Neurol 2000;47:606–13.

7. Reddy H, Narayanan S, Matthews PM, et al. Relating axonal injury to functional recovery in MS. Neurology 2000;54:236–9.

8. Reddy H, Narayanan S, Arnoutelis R, et al. Evidence for adaptive functional changes in the cerebral cortex with axonal injury from multiple sclerosis. Brain 2000;123:2314–20.

9. Werring DJ, Bullmore ET, Toosy AT, et al. Recovery from optic neuritis is associated with a change in the distribution of cerebral response to visual stimulation: a functional magnetic resonance imaging study. J Neurol Neurosurg Psychiatr 2000;68:441–9.

10. Langkilde AR, Frederiksen JL, Rostrup E, et al. Functional MRI of the visual cortex and visual testing in patients with previous optic neuritis. Eur J Neurol 2002;9:277–86.

11. Toosy AT, Werring DJ, Bullmore ET, et al. Functional magnetic resonance imaging of the cortical response to photic stimulation in humans following optic neuritis recovery. Neurosci Lett 2002;330:255–9.

12. Russ MO, Cleff U, Lanfermann H, et al. Functional magnetic resonance imaging in acute unilateral optic neuritis. J Neuroimaging 2002;12:339–50.

13. Toosy AT, Hickman SJ, Miszkiel KA, et al. Adaptive cortical plasticity in higher visual areas after acute optic neuritis. Ann Neurol 2005;57:622–33.

14. Levin N, Orlov T, Dotan S, et al. Normal and abnormal fMRI activation patterns in the visual cortex after recovery from optic neuritis. Neuroimage 2006;33:1161–8.

15. Korsholm K, Madsen KH, Frederiksen JL, et al. Recovery from optic neuritis: an ROI-based analysis of LGN and visual cortical areas. Brain 2007;130:1244–53.

16. Filippi M, Rocca MA, Falini A, et al. Correlations between structural CNS damage and functional MRI changes in primary progressive MS. Neuroimage 2002;15:537–46.

17. Rocca MA, Falini A, Colombo B, et al. Adaptive functional changes in the cerebral cortex of patients with non-disabling MS correlate with the extent of brain structural damage. Ann Neurol 2002;51:330–9.

18. Rocca MA, Mezzapesa DM, Falini A, et al. Evidence for axonal pathology and adaptive cortical reorganisation in patients at presentation with clinically isolated syndromes suggestive of MS. Neuroimage 2003;18:847–55.

19. Rocca MA, Gavazzi C, Mezzapesa DM, et al. A functional magnetic resonance imaging study of patients with secondary progressive multiple sclerosis. Neuroimage 2003;19:1770–7.

20. Rocca MA, Pagani E, Ghezzi A, et al. Functional cortical changes in patients with MS and non-specific conventional MRI scans of the brain. Neuroimage 2003;19:826–36.

21. Reddy H, Narayanan S, Woolrich M, et al. Functional brain reorganization for hand movement in patients with multiple sclerosis: defining distinct effects of injury and disability. Brain 2002;125:2646–57.

22. Filippi M, Rocca MA, Mezzapesa DM, et al. Simple and complex movement-associated functional MRI changes in patients at presentation with clinically isolated syndromes suggestive of MS. Hum Brain Mapp 2004;21:108–17.

23. Rocca MA, Mezzapesa DM, Ghezzi A, et al. A widespread pattern of cortical activations in patients at presentation with clinically isolated symptoms is associated with evolution to definite multiple sclerosis. AJNR Am J Neuroradiol 2005;26:1136–9.

24. Pantano P, Iannetti GD, Caramia F, et al. Cortical motor reorganization after a single clinical attack of multiple sclerosis. Brain 2002;125:1607–15.

25. Pantano P, Mainero C, Iannetti GD, et al. Contribution of corticospinal tract damage to cortical motor reorganization after a single clinical attack of multiple sclerosis. Neuroimage 2002;17:1837–43.

26. Rocca MA, Gallo A, Colombo B, et al. Pyramidal tract lesions and movement-associated cortical recruitment in patients with MS. Neuroimage 2004;23:141–7.

27. Lowe MJ, Phillips MD, Lurito JT, et al. Multiple sclerosis: low-frequency temporal blood oxygen level-dependent fluctuations indicate reduced functional connectivity initial results. Radiology 2002;224:184–92.

28. Rocca MA, Matthews PM, Caputo D, et al. Evidence for widespread movement-associated functional MRI changes in patients with PPMS. Neurology 2002;58:866–72.

29. Rocca MA, Mezzapesa DM, Ghezzi A, et al. Cord damage elicits brain functional reorganization after a single episode of myelitis. Neurology 2003;61:1078–85.

30. Lowe MJ, Beall EB, Sakaie KE, et al. Resting state sensorimotor functional connectivity in multiple sclerosis inversely correlates with transcallosal motor pathway transverse diffusivity. Hum Brain Mapp 2008;29:818–27.

31. Rocca MA, Colombo B, Falini A, et al. Cortical adaptation in patients with MS: a cross-sectional functional MRI study of disease phenotypes. Lancet Neurol 2005;4:618–26.

32. Rocca MA, Agosta F, Colombo B, et al. fMRI changes in relapsing-remitting multiple sclerosis patients complaining of fatigue after IFNβ-1a injection. Hum Brain Mapp 2007;28:373–82.

33. Mezzapesa DM, Rocca MA, Rodegher M, et al. Functional cortical changes of the sensorimotor network are associated with clinical recovery in multiple sclerosis. Hum Brain Mapp 2008;29:562–73.

34. Rocca MA, Tortorella P, Ceccarelli A, et al. The mirror-neuron system in MS: a 3 Tesla fMRI study. Neurology 2008;70:255–62.

35. Rocca MA, Pagani E, Absinta M, et al. Altered functional and structural connectivities in patients with MS: a 3T fMRI study. Neurology 2007;69: 2136–45.

36. Ciccarelli O, Toosy AT, Marsden JF, et al. Functional response to active and passive ankle movements with clinical correlations in patients with primary progressive multiple sclerosis. J Neurol 2006;253: 882–91.

37. Filippi M, Rocca MA, Mezzapesa DM, et al. A functional MRI study of cortical activations associated with object manipulation in patients with MS. Neuroimage 2004;21:1147–54.

38. Cerasa A, Fera F, Gioia MC, et al. Adaptive cortical changes and the functional correlates of visuo-motor integration in relapsing-remitting multiple sclerosis. Brain Res Bull 2006;69: 597–605.

39. Staffen W, Mair A, Zauner H, et al. Cognitive function and fMRI in patients with multiple sclerosis: evidence for compensatory cortical activation during an attention task. Brain 2002;125: 1275–82.

40. Au Duong MV, Audoin B, Boulanouar K, et al. Altered functional connectivity related to white matter changes inside the working memory network at the very early stage of MS. J Cereb Blood Flow Metab 2005;25:1245–53.

41. Au Duong MV, Boulanouar K, Audoin B, et al. Modulation of effective connectivity inside the working memory network in patients at the earliest stage of multiple sclerosis. Neuroimage 2005;24: 533–8.

42. Audoin B, Ibarrola D, Ranjeva JP, et al. Compensatory cortical activation observed by fMRI during a cognitive task at the earliest stage of MS. Hum Brain Mapp 2003;20:51–8.

43. Audoin B, Au Duong MV, Ranjeva JP, et al. Magnetic resonance study of the influence of tissue damage and cortical reorganization on PASAT performance at the earliest stage of multiple sclerosis. Hum Brain Mapp 2005;24:216–28.

44. Hillary FG, Chiaravalloti ND, Ricker JH, et al. An investigation of working memory rehearsal in multiple sclerosis using fMRI. J Clin Exp Neuropsychol 2003;25:965–78.

45. Parry AM, Scott RB, Palace J, et al. Potentially adaptive functional changes in cognitive processing for patients with multiple sclerosis and their acute modulation by rivastigmine. Brain 2003;126: 2750–60.

46. Penner IK, Rausch M, Kappos L, et al. Analysis of impairment related functional architecture in MS patients during performance of different attention tasks. J Neurol 2003;250:461–72.

47. Mainero C, Caramia F, Pozzilli C, et al. fMRI evidence of brain reorganization during attention and memory tasks in multiple sclerosis. Neuroimage 2004;21:858–67.

48. Sweet LH, Rao SM, Primeau M, et al. Functional magnetic resonance imaging of working memory among multiple sclerosis patients. J Neuroimaging 2004;14:150–7.

49. Sweet LH, Rao SM, Primeau M, et al. Functional magnetic resonance imaging response to increased verbal working memory demands among patients with multiple sclerosis. Hum Brain Mapp 2006;27: 28–36.

50. Wishart HA, Saykin AJ, McDonald BC, et al. Brain activation patterns associated with working memory in relapsing-remitting MS. Neurology 2004;62:234–8.

51. Chiaravalloti N, Hillary F, Ricker J, et al. Cerebral activation patterns during working memory performance in multiple sclerosis using FMRI. J Clin Exp Neuropsychol 2005;27:33–54.

52. Cader S, Cifelli A, Abu-Omar Y, et al. Reduced brain functional reserve and altered functional connectivity in patients with multiple sclerosis. Brain 2006; 129:527–37.

53. Li Y, Chiaravalloti ND, Hillary FG, et al. Differential cerebellar activation on functional magnetic resonance imaging during working memory performance in persons with multiple sclerosis. Arch Phys Med Rehabil 2004;85:635–9.

54. Rocca MA, Valsasina P, Ceccarelli A, et al. Structural and functional MRI correlates of Stroop control in benign MS. Hum Brain Mapp, in press.

55. Lazeron RH, Rombouts SA, Scheltens P, et al. An fMRI study of planning-related brain activity in patients with moderately advanced multiple sclerosis. Mult Scler 2004;10:549–55.

56. Stroman PW. Magnetic resonance imaging of neuronal function in the spinal cord: spinal FMRI. Clin Med Res 2005;3:146–56 [Review].

57. Agosta F, Valsasina P, Caputo D, et al. Tactile-associated fMRI recruitment of the cervical cord in healthy subjects. Hum Brain Mapp, in press.

58. Agosta F, Valsasina P, Rocca MA, et al. Evidence for enhanced functional activity of cervical cord in relapsing multiple sclerosis. Magn Reson Med 2008; 59:1035–42.

59. Agosta F, Valsasina P, Caputo D, et al. Tactile-associated recruitment of cervical cord is altered in patients with multiple sclerosis. Neuroimage 2008;39: 1542–8.

60. Lenzi D, Conte A, Mainero C, et al. Effect of corpus callosum damage on ipsilateral motor activation in patients with multiple sclerosis: a functional and anatomical study. Hum Brain Mapp 2007;28: 636–44.

61. Manson SC, Palace J, Frank JA, et al. Loss of interhemispheric inhibition in patients with multiple sclerosis is related to corpus callosum atrophy. Exp Brain Res 2006;174:728–33.

62. Pantano P, Mainero C, Lenzi D, et al. A longitudinal fMRI study on motor activity in patients with multiple sclerosis. Brain 2005;128:2146–53.

63. Mainero C, Inghilleri M, Pantano P, et al. Enhanced brain motor activity in patients with MS after a single dose of 3,4-diaminopyridine. Neurology 2004;62:2044–50.

64. Morgen K, Kadom N, Sawaki L, et al. Training-dependent plasticity in patients with multiple sclerosis. Brain 2004;127:2506–17.

65. Wegner C, Filippi M, Barkhof F, et al. Relating functional changes during hand movement to clinical parameters in patients with multiple sclerosis in a multi-centre fMRI study. Eur J Neurol 2008; 15:113–22.

66. Rocca MA, Absinta M, Valsasina P, et al. Abnormal connectivity of the sensorimotor network in patients with MS: a multi-centre fMRI study. Hum Brain Mapp 2008, in press.

Nonconventional Optic Nerve Imaging in Multiple Sclerosis

Christopher C. Glisson, DO, MS[a,b], Steven L. Galetta, MD[c],*

KEYWORDS

- Optic nerve • Neuroimaging
- Optic coherence tomography
- Diffusion weighted MR imaging
- Magnetization transfer MR imaging • Multiple sclerosis

Multiple sclerosis (MS) is a disease characterized by demyelination and axonal injury,[1] disseminated in time and space. Definitive diagnosis requires the documentation of discrete clinical events, with neurologic symptoms or neuroimaging studies demonstrating involvement of different areas within the central nervous system (CNS). Over time, it has been recognized that a significant degree of discordance exists between radiographic lesions and clinical disability. Therefore, the link between structure (as assessed by conventional imaging techniques) and function is incomplete. Moreover, it is logical to infer from this observation that the progression of MS is, in large part, subclinical, further emphasizing the need for novel means of detecting disease evolution in susceptible individuals.

Despite significant variability in the clinical presentation of MS, vision loss attributable to acute demyelinating optic neuritis (ON) is often the initial manifestation.[2–4] Similarly, MS is thought to be the most common cause of ON. Unfortunately, an episode of ON is not sufficient to diagnose MS; indeed, some patients will recover and never again develop neurologic symptoms. A particular challenge remains unsolved: how to identify those patients with ON who will subsequently develop MS, and, once identified, how to longitudinally monitor them to ensure clinical stability. Thus far, conventional neuroimaging techniques (including magnetic resonance imaging [MR imaging]) have been used in conjunction with clinical measures to determine the risk of developing MS for patients with ON. As a consequence of these investigations, much has been learned about the pathophysiology, and the natural history, by which these two conditions are associated.

Unique features of the optic nerve, including its frequent involvement early in the course of MS, and the relative ease by which both structure and function can be analyzed, make the anterior visual pathway a compelling model for the evaluation of inflammatory-demyelinating disease elsewhere within the central nervous system (CNS). It has now been established that patients with MS manifest subclinical alterations in optic nerve function;[5] these dynamic changes lend themselves to longitudinal monitoring.

Seeking to capitalize on the accessibility and vulnerability of the optic nerve in MS, various nonconventional imaging techniques have been developed. As with any structural assessment, effective implementation requires validation by reliable and useful clinical outcomes. Through the correlation of these novel imaging strategies with established measures of anterior visual pathway

a Department of Neurology and Ophthalmology, Michigan State University College of Human Medicine, 260 Jefferson SE, Suite 217, Grand Rapids, MI 49503, USA
b Neuro-Ophthalmology, Saint Mary's Health Care, Grand Rapids, Michigan, USA
c Division of Neuro-Ophthalmology, Department of Neurology, University of Pennsylvania School of Medicine, 3 East Gates Building, 3400 Spruce Street, Philadelphia, PA 19104, USA
* Corresponding author. Division of Neuro-Ophthalmology, Department of Neurology, University of Pennsylvania School of Medicine, 3 East Gates Building, 3400 Spruce Street, Philadelphia, PA 19104.
E-mail address: Steve.Galetta@uphs.upenn.edu (S.L. Galetta).

Neuroimag Clin N Am 19 (2009) 71–79
doi:10.1016/j.nic.2008.09.003

function, advances in the early detection and serial monitoring of demyelinating disease are rapidly emerging. Moreover, the opportunity to assess here-to-fore unseen changes as a result of disease evolution allows for more sensitive analysis of the efficacy of candidate neuroprotective agents.

Specific quantitative imaging techniques relevant to the optic nerve include measurement of optic nerve atrophy, magnetization transfer (MT) MR imaging, diffusion tensor (DT) MR imaging, and optical coherence tomography (OCT).

OPTIC NERVE ANATOMY

The paired optic nerves, each 50 mm in length, serve to transmit visual information from the retina to the optic chiasm. Each optic nerve, from the globe to the chiasm, is composed of four parts: *intraocular* (optic nerve head, 1 mm), *intraorbital* (25 mm), *intracanalicular* (traversing the optic canal, 9 mm), and *intracranial* (stretching from the canal to the optic chiasm, 4 to 16 mm). Each is composed of a bundle of nerve fibers that maintain a topical arrangement along their course from the retina through the optic chiasm. The optic nerves are, histologically and phylogenetically, extensions of brain, and are surrounded by cerebrospinal fluid (CSF). These unique characteristics allow the optic nerve to serve as a model for disease processes occurring elsewhere within the CNS, including demyelination and axonal loss.

OPTIC NEURITIS: CLINICAL PRESENTATION

In the absence of other symptoms of MS, acute demyelinating ON is referred to as one of the clinically isolated syndromes (CIS) suggestive of MS. Young to middle-aged persons (second through fourth decade) are most commonly affected. ON is approximately three times more common in women than in men.[3,6,7] Patients present with vision loss that is acute or subacute. In greater than 90% of patients, pain exacerbated by eye movements is reported. The degree of vision loss is variable, with median visual acuity of 20/60 at presentation. Most patients improve within several weeks of onset.[6,8] The clinical examination should disclose the presence of an afferent pupillary defect. In two thirds of the patients, optic nerve appearance will be normal.[9] Almost any visual field defect can occur, although central scotoma or diffuse field loss is the most common.[10] If visual function worsens beyond a 2-week period, or does not improve within 4 weeks, alternate etiologies should be considered.[7,9,11] Improvement in acuity can be hastened through the use of intravenous corticosteroids.[11] Other aspects of vision, including color perception, low-contrast letter acuity, and depth perception, often remain deficient. Uhthoff's phenomenon (a transient worsening of vision following exercise or exposure to heat) may occur.

CONVENTIONAL MR IMAGING: LESIONS OF THE OPTIC NERVE

The diagnosis of acute, monosymptomatic ON is often based on the appropriate clinical history and supportive examination findings, without the need for neuroimaging. However, data from the Optic Neuritis Treatment Trial (ONTT)[12] and the Longitudinal Optic Neuritis Study (LONS)[13,14] have highlighted the utility of brain MR imaging in predicting the subsequent risk of developing MS. In atypical cases, MR imaging of the orbits should be obtained to exclude an alternate diagnosis, such as a compressive lesion.

In acute monophasic ON, the most effective conventional MR imaging sequences are (1) short tau inversion recovery (STIR), (2) fast spin-echo (FSE) T2-weighted images, and (3) spin-echo T1 pre- and post-gadolinium fat-suppressed sequences.[15–17] With these techniques, the causative lesion can frequently be identified (**Fig. 1**). Typical findings include dilation of the optic nerve sheath immediately posterior to the globe on fat-saturated FSE sequences, and optic nerve sheath enhancement (a high-signal ring corresponding to the optic nerve sheath) on gadolinium-enhanced images. Although previously thought rare in patients with acute ON, a study by Hickman and colleagues[18] has suggested that optic nerve sheath dilatation (45%) and optic nerve sheath enhancement (75%) are common findings. However, these findings are nonspecific, and cannot distinguish ON from ischemic or infectious causes of optic neuropathy. Moreover, collective clinical and experimental evidence has repeatedly shown a poor correlation between MS lesions detected by conventional MR imaging, and functional disability.[19–22] Therefore, the use of MR imaging as an outcome metric for assessing disease progression, and response to disease modifying therapies, is imperfect. It is because of these and other limitations that the development of nonconventional imaging techniques has become necessary.

OPTIC NERVE ATROPHY

While classically considered an inflammatory-demyelinating process, both acute and chronic phases of MS have been shown to result in axonal injury;[1] this is the basis for progressive and permanent neurologic dysfunction as a consequence of

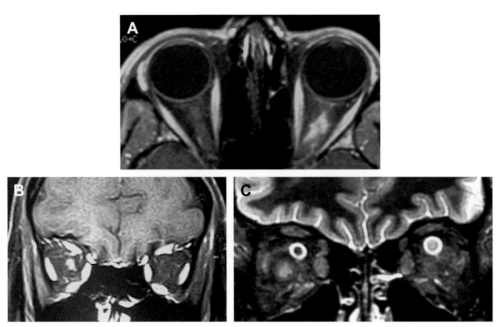

Fig. 1. (A) Axial T1-weighted MR image demonstrating gadolinium enhancement of the left optic nerve in acute optic neuritis. (B) T1-weighted coronal MR image with enhancement of the optic nerve sheath in acute optic neuritis. (C) T2-weighted coronal image from a patient with optic neuritis showing increased signal intensity in the optic nerve.

demyelinating disease. Following the acute phase of ON (when the inflammatory process results in edema of the optic nerve), ongoing demyelination results in axon loss and atrophy. This process was first documented using conventional optic nerve imaging in patients with ON.[23] With more recent improvements in MR imaging techniques, including fat- and CSF-suppressed sequences, analysis of optic nerve atrophy has been reliably correlated with functional impairment. Hickman and colleagues[24] described a fat-saturated short echo fast fluid-attenuated inversion-recovery (sTE fFLAIR) sequence to overcome the high signal from orbital fat and CSF surrounding the optic nerve. Using this technique, an in-plane resolution of 0.5 mm^2 and 3-mm slice thickness was achieved, allowing for the measurement of optic nerve atrophy following a single episode of ON. Equally important was the observation that the degree of atrophy was related to disease duration, further underscoring the impact of ongoing axonal degeneration as a consequence of demyelination. Progressive atrophy was associated with poor visual recovery and reduced visual evoked potential (VEP) amplitude.[25] In yet another series of 21 patients, mean optic nerve diameter in eyes with acute ON was reduced compared with contralateral eyes and healthy controls.[26] These data suggest that measurement of optic nerve atrophy may be a useful strategy for determining the stage of ON, and for following axonal loss over time.

MAGNETIZATION TRANSFER MR IMAGING

Magnetization transfer MR imaging (MT MR imaging) provides an analysis of the degree of tissue damage, both within and surrounding demyelinating lesions. By measuring macromolecular density, MT MR imaging is superior to conventional MR imaging in its specificity for detecting irreversible demyelination and axonal injury. The studies completed to date suggest that MT MR imaging correlates with functional outcome measures, and may be a useful technique for the longitudinal monitoring of patients with MS.

The principle of MT MR imaging[27,28] is predicated on differences in the interactions of free and bound protons when exposed to off-resonance irradiation. The magnetization of bound protons becomes saturated; these protons then transfer magnetization to more mobile protons, resulting in reduction of the tissue signal. The difference in signal intensity before and after the pulse allows for calculation of the MT ratio (MTR); a low MTR is indicative of tissue damage resulting from demyelination and axon loss. Conversely, recovery of MTR may reflect remyelination, or resolution of acute inflammation/edema.[29] In a serial imaging study of four patients with MS,[30] decreases in MTR were most promi-nent at lesion appearance, and during the first 2 months thereafter. Of the 15 lesions docu-mented, MTR then returned to normal in five of them, and eight showed a slower rate of decline over subsequent months. These findings suggest that normalization of MTR is attributable to resolv-ing edema, while progressive declines may be a marker of further demyelination and axonal loss. As an additional confirmatory measure, values obtained by MTR have been correlated with axonal injury and conventional MR lesions through postmortem studies.[31,32]

Once again, application of this imaging strategy in ON has yielded compelling in vivo data docu-menting the initial and longitudinal effects of MS. In 39 patients with acute ON,[33] the mean intraorbi-tal MTR measured 30.6 percent units (pu) in optic nerves demonstrating either a high-signal T2 lesion or contrast enhancement, compared with 41.1 pu in healthy controls. In another study,[29] 20 patients analyzed between 3 months and 16 years after a course of unilateral ON were similarly found to have decreased mean MTR in the affected intraorbital optic nerve when compared with the contralateral optic nerve and healthy controls. The reduction in MTR was found to be inversely correlated with VEP latency, suggesting a relationship between decreased MTR and demy-elination. Another cohort of patients with prior ON demonstrated a correlation between MTR and visual acuity.[34]

To overcome the limitations of two-dimensional gradient-echo imaging (specifically, the need for manual placement of a region-of-interest [ROI] of 4 to 8 voxels that may exclude data if the optic nerves are swollen, or include partial-volume pixels containing CSF or orbital fat if the optic nerves are atrophic), Hickman and colleagues[35] used a high-resolution gradient echo sequence to prospectively evaluate optic nerve MTR in a cohort of patients with acute unilateral ON. At the onset of symptoms, when vision was most af-fected, MTR values were unchanged (compared with acute brain lesions, which demonstrate a rapid initial decrease in MTR). This finding was attributed to two factors: in the initial stages fol-lowing axonal transection, Wallerian degeneration may increase MTR as a result of increased expo-sure of myelin fragments. In addition, structural features limiting the development of vasogenic edema in the optic nerve may lessen the effect of blood–optic nerve barrier breakdown on MTR. During the period of visual recovery, mean MTR continued to decline until reaching a nadir at approximately 8 months. This finding, the authors suggest, indicates that there are factors involved

in visual recovery that are not detected by MTR, and that tissue changes within the optic nerve con-tinue for several months following the initial ON event, and following visual recovery. Finally, lower time-averaged MTRs were associated with worse visual outcomes.

MT MR imaging is emerging as another noncon-ventional MR strategy to circumvent the barrier of discordance between MR imaging appearance and neurologic dysfunction. Furthermore, MTR can be measured in different segments along the whole of the optic nerve, thus providing informa-tion concerning the progressive nature of demye-lination and remyelination over time. This particular feature is of potential value as the effects of disease-modifying therapies are evaluated.

DIFFUSION TENSOR MR IMAGING

Advances in image acquisition and post-process-ing have allowed the use of DT MR imaging in the longitudinal study of patients with MS. As with other quantitative MR imaging techniques, it is noninvasive and can both detect and quantify tissue changes within and around demyelinating lesions. Application of this technique allows for quantification of the structural integrity of axons; as a result, DT MR imaging represents another potential surrogate for monitoring disease pro-gression in MS.

The principle of DT MR imaging[36] is based on *diffusion*, defined as the random translational movement of molecules within a fluid system. The effect of intact CNS tissue components is to make the MR imaging-measured diffusion coeffi-cient lower than that in free water; this is termed the apparent diffusion coefficient (ADC, **Fig. 2**). Injury to CNS tissues (for example, demyelination or axonal damage) results in an increase in ADC. As the magnitude of diffusion is dependent on the direction of measurement, application of a matrix to account for the correlation of molecular displacement along orthogonal directions allows for complete analysis of the diffusion pattern (**Fig. 3**). From this, specific values known as mean diffusivity (MD) and fractional anisotropy (FA) can be derived.

Demyelination within the optic nerve (as in cere-bral white matter) is associated with increases in MD and reductions in FA. These differences can be quantified, and have been shown to correlate with disability in patients with both relapsing-remitting and secondary-progressive MS.[37] This technique can be further applied to the optic nerve, providing an additional outcome measure for the detection of early structural alterations in

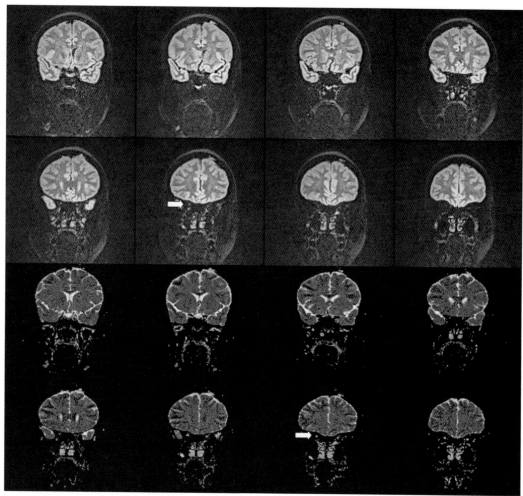

Fig. 2. Diffusion-weighted (DW) MR image with Periodically Rotated Overlapping ParallEL Lines with Enhanced Reconstruction (PROPELLER) data acquisition for optic nerve evaluation. Appearance of the optic nerve (arrows) in a healthy volunteer using DW MR imaging and apparent diffusion coefficient (ADC) maps. (*Courtesy of* Elias R. Melhem, MD, PhD, Philadelphia, PA.)

ON, or to follow changes with time as a result of therapy.

Application of this technique first required the development of a fat- and CSF-suppressed zonal oblique multislice echo planar imaging (ZOOM-EPI) diffusion-weighted sequence, to allow detection of increases in ADC following ON.[38,39] Using this novel technique, 25 patients with unilateral ON in the previous year were compared with 15 healthy controls.[40] Non–diffusion-weighted images were used to segment the intraorbital optic nerves, and ROI were transferred to MD and FA maps for quantitative analysis. When compared with unaffected contralateral and control optic nerves, mean MD was significantly elevated and mean FA significantly reduced in eyes with ON. While there was no correlation with clinical measures of visual function, DT MR imaging

parameters did correlate with changes in whole-field VEP. Thus far, DT MR imaging of the optic nerve has been limited by the large amount of orbital bone that surrounds the optic nerve and the artifact that results from magnetic signal inhomogeneity in this region.

In brain studies, DT MR imaging has been shown to detect the pathologic changes of demyelination and axonal loss before lesions become visible by conventional MR imaging.[41] Furthermore, DT MR imaging may have the capacity to assess the severity of disease progression as a function of axonal loss.[42] Finally, longitudinal evaluations of patients with MS using DT MR imaging have shown that it is sensitive to subtle changes over short time intervals,[22,43] further enhancing its utility in the serial monitoring of disease.

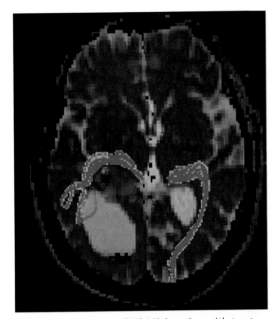

Fig. 3. Diffusion tensor (DT) MR imaging with tractography of the optic tracts from the lateral geniculate nuclei to occipital cortex. Tracts on the right are displaced by an intra-ventricular meningioma. (*Courtesy of* Elias R. Melhem, MD, PhD, Philadelphia, PA.)

The implications of these observations, and their extrapolation to ongoing studies of the optic nerve in MS, cannot be overstated: as previously discussed, changes within the optic nerve are often present early, and an imaging modality with the ability to detect the pathologic features underlying demyelination and axonal injury holds tremendous promise for understanding disease progression. As a surrogate marker of the structural integrity of optic nerve axons, DT MR imaging offers the opportunity for in vivo analysis of disease activity, and potentially represents a useful tool for monitoring the response to a number of therapies.

OPTICAL COHERENCE TOMOGRAPHY

As a technique for detecting subtle but important tissue changes brought about as a consequence of demyelinating disease, OCT has received significant attention. OCT allows for the direct visualization of the relevant tissues themselves; thus, the integrity of the optic nerve fibers as they originate from the retinal ganglion cells can be assessed. OCT circumvents the barrier of the skull, providing a "window" into the disease process and a reflection of alterations occurring elsewhere in the CNS.[44,45] The theoretic utility of OCT is predicated on the recognition of atrophy of the inner retinal layers[46] and optic nerve in MS. As a diagnostic modality, it is inexpensive (10% to 15% of the cost of conventional MR imaging), noninvasive, fast, accurate, and reproducible.

In a manner similar to B-scan ultrasonography (but using light instead of sound), OCT employs a super-luminescent diode to project a broadband near-infrared light beam centered at 820 nm onto the retina. Reflection delay and backscattering of light is compared with a reference reflection by an optical interferometer. Over 1000 data points distributed over 2 mm in depth are sampled; the data are then used to reconstruct a cross-sectional image of the retinal anatomy, which can be evaluated both quantitatively and qualitatively (**Fig. 4**).

Numerous studies have been undertaken to validate the performance of OCT in measuring the thickness of the retinal nerve fiber layer (RNFL) and macular volume (MV),[47,48] and in detecting RNFL thinning (due to axon damage) in the retinas of patients with MS. Importantly, OCT is sensitive to changes in RNFL even in patients without a clinical history of ON,[45,49,50] further emphasizing the potential of OCT for using the anterior visual pathway as a model for demyelination elsewhere within the CNS.

OCT has also been correlated with changes detected on conventional MR imaging in patients with MS. A cross-sectional, case-control study[51] of 40 patients with MS and 15 controls found a significant association between RNFL thinning and global brain atrophy (assessed by increased CSF volume). Using a 3.0-Tesla scanner, anatomic MR imaging data were acquired using a magnetization-prepared rapid gradient echo (MPRAGE) protocol. Brain tissue volumes were then normalized for subject head size, and a measure of whole brain atrophy (brain parenchymal fraction, BPF) calculated. Minimum RNFL thickness, as well as age, was found to predict a significant amount of variance in BPF and CSF volume.

As further evidence of the ability of OCT to detect subclinical changes in RNFL and MV, 163 patients with MS and 47 control subjects were imaged in an outpatient neurology clinic setting.[52] Visual function testing was performed in 296 MS eyes and 64 control eyes using low-contrast Sloan letter charts. Low-contrast letter acuity is an emerging outcome measure for clinical trials in MS, given its ability to reliably distinguish patients with MS from disease-free controls.[53–55] The average RNFL thickness was reduced in patients with a clinical history of ON (84.2 ± 14.7 mm) compared with healthy controls (102.7 ± 11.5 mm). Patients with MS but no history of ON also demonstrated decreased RNFL thickness (95.9 ± 14 mm). Unaffected eyes of patients with unilateral MS also had a decrease in RNFL (93.9 ± 13.1 mm). RNFL

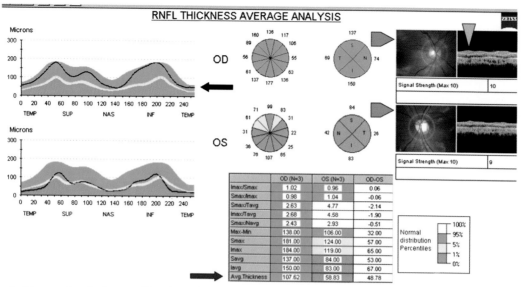

	OD (N=3)	OS (N=3)	OD-OS
Imax/Smax	1.02	0.96	0.06
Smax/Imax	0.98	1.04	-0.06
Smax/Tavg	2.63	4.77	-2.14
Imax/Tavg	2.68	4.58	-1.90
Smax/Navg	2.43	2.93	-0.51
Max-Min	138.00	106.00	32.00
Smax	181.00	124.00	57.00
Imax	184.00	119.00	65.00
Savg	137.00	84.00	53.00
Iavg	150.00	83.00	67.00
Avg.Thickness	107.62	58.83	48.78

Fig. 4. Abnormal retinal nerve fiber layer (RNFL) thickness report showing the optical coherence tomography (OCT) images, fundus images, and thickness charts/plots for each eye of a patient with multiple sclerosis (MS). This patient had a history of acute optic neuritis in each eye, and a 7-year history of relapsing-remitting MS. The OCT 3 imager scans the peripapillary retina in a circular motion as shown in the fundus image (*red arrow*), producing an average RNFL thickness for the entire circumference (average thickness, in microns, *blue arrow*) as well as thickness values for the temporal, superior, nasal, and inferior retinal quadrants (*circular diagrams and thickness charts*) and for 12 clock hours. The RNFL is the innermost retinal layer on the two-dimensional cross-sectional image (depicted as top orange layer [*marked by orange arrow*]). Graphs show whether actual thickness values for the subject's eye (*black line indicated by black arrow*) fall outside the 5th and the 95th percentiles for age (values in yellow [below 5th percentile] and in red zones [below 1st percentile] on thickness plots) based on normative data included in the OCT software. (*Courtesy of* Laura J. Balcer, MD, MSCE, Philadelphia, PA.)

thickness was found to correlate with MS subtypes: patients with the progressive forms of MS had a more marked decrease in RNFL than patients with relapsing-remitting MS when compared with controls. Furthermore, visual acuity testing correlated with RNFL thickness values, suggesting that OCT may have clinical relevance as a measure of structural change related to MS.

Given that it is axon loss, and not demyelination, that underlies permanent clinical disability in MS, it is likely that the ability of OCT to accurately and reproducibly detect subclinical damage within the optic nerve will provide an effective biomarker of destructive disease elsewhere in the CNS.[56,57] Furthermore, retinal nerve fiber layer thickness and macular volume analysis may be reasonable outcome metrics for evaluating the neuroprotective effects of novel therapies in MS.

SUMMARY

It is well recognized that conventional MR imaging is, at present, the most important paraclinical modality for assessing the risk of MS in patients with acute demyelinating ON, and for monitoring the progression of disease. However, there are several limitations that limit the utility of conventional MR in imaging the optic nerve. Furthermore, conventional MR imaging is inadequate as an outcome metric for clinical trials of neuroprotective agents. Newer strategies, including measurement of optic atrophy, MT MR imaging, DT MR imaging, and OCT, show significant promise. Future investigations, including the use of nonconventional MR imaging techniques coupled with OCT and functional measures of anterior visual pathway function, will further assist in the early detection of clinical impairment. Serial analysis will allow for monitoring of disease progression, predict accumulation of disability, and ascertain the effects of candidate neuroprotective therapies.

REFERENCES

1. Trapp BD, Peterson J, Ransohoff RM, et al. Axonal transaction of the lesions of multiple sclerosis. N Engl J Med 1998;338:1268–76.
2. Balcer LJ, Galetta SL. Optic neuritis. In: Rakel RE, Bope ET, editors. Conn's current therapy. Philadelphia: WB Saunders; 2004. p. 187–90.
3. Balcer LJ. Optic neuritis. N Engl J Med 2006;354:43–50.

4. Arnold AC. Evolving management of optic neuritis and multiple sclerosis. Am J Ophthalmol 2005;139:1101–8.
5. Frohman EM, Frohman TC, Zee DS, et al. Neuro-ophthalmology of multiple sclerosis. Lancet Neurol 2005;4:111–21.
6. Beck RW. The optic neuritis treatment trial. Arch Ophthalmol 1988;106:151–3.
7. Liu GT. Visual loss: optic neuropathies. In: Liu GT, Volpe NJ, Galetta SL, editors. Neuro-ophthalmology: diagnosis and management. Philadelphia: WB Saunders; 2000. p.103–87.
8. Beck RW, Cleary PA, Backlund J, et al. The course of visual recovery after optic neuritis: experience of the optic neuritis treatment trial. Ophthalmology 1993;101:1771–8.
9. Optic neuritis study group. The clinical profile of acute optic neuritis: experience of the optic neuritis treatment trial. Arch Ophthalmol 1991;109:1673–8.
10. Keltner JL, Johnson CA, Spurr JO, et al. Baseline visual field profile of optic neuritis: the experience of the Optic Neuritis Treatment Trial. Arch Ophthalmol 1993;111:231–4.
11. Kaufman DI, Trobe JD, Eggenberger ER, et al. Practice parameter: the role of corticosteroids in the management of acute monosymptomatic optic neuritis. Report of the Quality Standards Subcommittee of the American Academy of Neurology. Neurology 2000;54:2039–44.
12. Beck RW, Arington J, Murtaugh FR, et al. Brain MRI in acute optic neuritis: experience of the Optic Neuritis Study Group. Arch Neurol 1993;8:841–6.
13. Optic neuritis study group. Visual function more than 10 years after optic neuritis: experience of the optic neuritis treatment trial. Am J Ophthalmol 2004;137(1):77–83.
14. Optic neuritis study group. Visual function 15 years after optic neuritis: a final follow-up report of from the optic neuritis treatment trial. Ophthalmology 2007;10.1016/j.ophtha.2007.08.004.
15. Gass A, Moseley AF, Barker GJ, et al. Lesion discrimination in optic neuritis using high-resolution fat-supressed fast spin-echo MRI. Neuroradiology 1996;38:317–21.
16. Kupersmith MJ, Alban T, Zeiffer B, et al. Contrast-enhanced MRI in acute optic neuritis: relationship to visual performance. Brain 2002;125:812–22.
17. Hickman SJ, Toosey AT, Miszkiel KA, et al. Visual recovery following acute optic neuritis: a clinical, electrophysiological and magnetic resonance imaging study. J Neurol 2004;251:996–1005.
18. Hickman SJ, Miszkiel KA, Plant GT, et al. The optic nerve sheath on MRI in acute optic neuritis. Neuroradiology 2005;47:51–5.
19. Brex PA, Ciccarelli O, O'Riordan JI, et al. A longitudinal study of abnormalities on MRI and disability from multiple sclerosis. N Engl J Med 2002;346:158–64.
20. Rovaris M, Filippi M, Falautano M, et al. Relation between MR abnormalities and patterns of cognitive impairment in multiple sclerosis. Neurology 1998;50:1601–8.
21. van Walderveen MA, Lycklama à Nijeholt GJ, Ader HJ, et al. Hypointense lesions on T1-weighted spin-echo magnetic resonance imaging: relation to clinical characteristics in subgroups of patients with multiple sclerosis. Arch Neurol 2001;58:76–81.
22. Rovaris M, Gallo A, Valsasina P, et al. Short-term accrual of gray matter pathology in patients with progressive multiple sclerosis: an in vivo study using diffusion tensor MRI. Neuroimage 2005;24:1139–46.
23. Youl BD, Turano G, Towell AD, et al. Optic neuritis: swelling and atrophy. Electroencephalogr Clin Neurophysiol Suppl 1996;46:173–9.
24. Hickman SJ, Brex PA, Brierly CMH, et al. Detection of optic nerve atrophy following a single episode of unilateral optic neuritis by MRI, using a fat saturated short echo fast FLAIR sequence. Neuroradiology 2001;43:123–8.
25. Hickman SJ, Brierly CMH, Brex PA, et al. Continuing optic nerve atrophy following optic neuritis: a serial MRI study. Mult Scler 2002;8:339–42.
26. Hickman SJ, Toosy AT, Jones SJ, et al. A serial MRI study following optic nerve mean area in acute optic neuritis. Brain 2004;127:2498–505.
27. Wolff SD, Balaban RS. Magnetization transfer imaging: practical aspects and clinical applications. Radiology 1994;192:593–9.
28. Filippi M, Agosta F. Magnetization transfer MRI in multiple sclerosis. J Neuroimaging 2007;17:22S–6S.
29. Thorpe JW, Barker GJ, Jones SJ, et al. Magnetization transfer ratios and transverse magnetization decay curves in optic neuritis: correlation with clinical and electrophysiology. J Neurol Neurosurg Psychiatry 1995;59:487–92.
30. Dousset V, Gayou A, Brochet B, et al. Early structural changes in acute MS lesions assessed by serial magnetization transfer studies. Neurology 1998;51:1150–5.
31. van Waesberghe JH, Kamphorst W, De Groot C, et al. Axonal loss in multiple sclerosis lesions: magnetic resonance imaging insights into substrates of disability. Ann Neurol 1999;46:747–54.
32. Schmierer K, Scaravelli F, Altmann DR, et al. Magnetization transfer ratio and myelin in postmortem multiple sclerosis brain. Ann Neurol 2004;56:407–15.
33. Boorstein JM, Moonis G, Boorstein SM, et al. Optic neuritis: imaging with magnetization transfer. Am J Roentgenol 1997;169:1709–12.
34. Inglese M, Ghezzi A, Bianchi S, et al. Irreversible disability and tissue loss in multiple sclerosis: a conventional and magnetization transfer magnetic resonance imaging study of the optic nerves. Arch Neurol 2002;59:250–5.

35. Hickman SJ, Toosy AT, Jones SJ, et al. Serial magnetization transfer imaging in acute optic neuritis. Brain 2004;127:692–700.
36. Rovaris M, Filippi M. Diffusion tensor MRI in multiple sclerosis. J Neuroimaging 2007;17:27S–30S.
37. Cercignani M, Inglese M, Pagani E, et al. Mean diffusivity and fractional anisotropy histograms of patients with multiple sclerosis. Am J Neuroradiol 2001;22(5):952–8.
38. Hickman SJ. Optic nerve imaging in multiple sclerosis. J Neuroimaging 2007;17:42S–5S.
39. Hickman SJ, Wheeler-Kingshott CAM, Jones SJ. Optic nerve diffusion measurement from diffusion weighted imaging in optic neuritis. Am J Neuroradiol 2005;26:951–6.
40. Tripp SA, Wheeler-Kingshott CAM, Jones SJ, et al. Optic nerve diffusion tensor imaging in optic neuritis. Neuroimage 2006;30:498–505.
41. Rocca MA, Cercignani M, Iannucci G, et al. Weekly diffusion-weighted imaging of normal-appearing white matter in MS. Neurology 2000;55:882–4.
42. Bozzali M, Falini A, Franceschi M, et al. White matter damage in Alzheimer's disease assessed in vivo using diffusion tensor magnetic resonance imaging. J Neurol Neurosurg Psychiatry 2002;72:742–6.
43. Oreja-Guevara C, Rovaris M, Iannucci G, et al. Progressive gray matter damage in patients with relapsing-remitting MS: a longitudinal diffusion tensor MRI study. Arch Neurol 2005;62(4):578–84.
44. Miller N, Drachman DA. The optic nerve: a window into diseases of the brain? Neurology 2006;67:1742–3.
45. Frohman E, Costello F, Zivadinov R, et al. Optical coherence tomography in multiple sclerosis. Lancet Neurol 2006;5:853–63.
46. Kerrison JB, Flynn T, Green WR. Retinal pathologic changes in multiple sclerosis. Retina 1994;14:445–51.
47. Paunescu LA, Schuman JS, Price LL, et al. Reproducibility of nerve fiber thickness, macular thickness, and optic nerve head measurements using StratusOCT. Invest Ophthalmol Vis Sci 2004;45:1716–24.
48. Hee MR, Izatt JA, Swanson EA, et al. Optical coherence tomography of the human retina. Arch Ophthalmol 1995;113:325–32.
49. Fisher JB, Jacobs DA, Markowitz CE, et al. Relation of visual function to retinal nerve fiber layer thickness in multiple sclerosis. Ophthalmology 2006;113:324–32.
50. Costello F, Coupland S, Hodge W, et al. Quantifying axonal loss after optic neuritis with optical coherence tomography. Ann Neurol 2006;59:963–9.
51. Gordon-Lipkin E, Chodkowski B, Reich DS, et al. Retinal nerve fiber layer is associated with brain atrophy in multiple sclerosis. Neurology 2007;69:1603–9.
52. Pulicken M, Gordon-Lipkin E, Balcer LJ, et al. Optical coherence tomography and disease subtype in multiple sclerosis. Neurology 2007;69:2085–92.
53. Balcer LJ, Baier ML, Pelak VS, et al. New low-contrast vision charts: reliability and test characteristics in patients with multiple sclerosis. Mult Scler 2000;6:163–71.
54. Baier ML, Cutter GR, Rudnick RA, et al. Low-contrast letter acuity testing captures visual dysfunction in patients with multiple sclerosis. Neurology 2005;64:992–5.
55. Balcer LJ, Baier ML, Cohen JA, et al. Contrast letter acuity as a visual component for Multiple Sclerosis Functional Composite. Neurology 2003;61:1367–73.
56. Trip SA, Schlottmann PG, Jones SJ, et al. Retinal nerve fiber layer axonal loss and visual dysfunction in optic neuritis. Ann Neurol 2005;58:383–91.
57. Trip SA, Schlottmann PG, Jones SJ, et al. Optic nerve atrophy and retinal nerve fiber layer thinning following optic neuritis: evidence that axonal loss is a substrate of MRI-detected atrophy. Neuroimage 2006;31:286–93.

Spinal-Cord MRI in Multiple Sclerosis: Conventional and Nonconventional MR Techniques

Joseph CJ. Bot, MD, PhD*, Frederik Barkhof, MD, PhD

KEYWORDS

- Multiple sclerosis • Magnetic resonance imaging
- Spinal cord • Atrophy • DWI • Spectroscopy
- Functional MRI • Demyelination

The presence of hyperintense T2 lesions in the brain is a completely nonspecific finding, and many other autoimmune mediated inflammatory disorders (OID) and cerebrovascular diseases are known to produce brain lesions that may mimic multiple sclerosis (MS) on T2-weighted MRI. Multifocal areas of high signal intensity within the cerebral white matter with or without similar areas in the immediate periventricular region also may be seen on T2-weighted MRI in neurologically healthy people. The incidence of white matter abnormalities in the brain increases with age, and studies reported a prevalence of more than 30% in patients over the age of 60.[1] Differential diagnosis between MS and OID or cerebrovascular disease can be difficult on T2-weighted brain examinations, especially if patients also show clinical signs of central nervous system (CNS) involvement.[2]

Initial MR diagnostic criteria for MS were based on cerebral MR without inclusion of spinal cord MRI findings. These criteria were based on size, number, contrast enhancement, and location of focal abnormalities.[3–5] The accuracy of these criteria was far from optimal, which resulted in a substantial number of misclassifications in a diagnostic setting.[5,6] The spinal cord is frequently involved in MS, with more than 90% of patients who have MS showing abnormalities on T2-weighted MRI. In contrast to the brain, MS-like abnormalities are seldom found in the spinal cord of healthy volunteers, even past 50 years of age.[1,7] Although spinal cord abnormalities have been reported in OID and cerebrovascular disease, appearance of such abnormalities may differ from those seen in MS.[8–18] Spinal cord MRI may therefore be of great value, in addition to brain MRI, for the differential diagnosis of MS.[8,9]

This article addresses conventional and quantitative techniques for spinal cord MRI in patients who have MS, their relation to clinical and histopathologic variables, and the diagnostic value of spinal cord MRI within the McDonald criteria for MS.

Search strategy and selection criteria: Data for this review were identified by searches of MEDLINE with the terms "multiple sclerosis", "magnetic resonance imaging", "spinal cord", "atrophy", "DWI", "spectroscopy", "functional MRI" and "demyelination". Further, articles identified through searches of the files of the authors, and through references cited in the articles were used. Only papers published in English were reviewed. Precise information on unpublished or in-press data was obtained through personal communication with researchers who work in the same research groups as the authors. In clinical work-up of clinically isolated syndrome patients imaging of the spinal cord has become a useful tool.
Department of Radiology, MR Center for MS Research, VU Medical Center, 1007 MB Amsterdam, The Netherlands
* Corresponding author.
E-mail address: j.bot@vumc.nl (J.CJ. Bot).

Neuroimag Clin N Am 19 (2009) 81–99
doi:10.1016/j.nic.2008.09.005

TECHNICAL FEATURES: WHICH SEQUENCE TO USE

Imaging of the spinal cord in an adequate fashion is one of the most challenging features in MRI because images may be influenced by many sources of artifacts. Because of the location within the spinal canal, motion of the thorax, heart, and spinal cord, and additional turbulent and pulsatile flow of surrounding cerebrospinal fluid (CSF), ghosting artifacts, truncation artifacts, and patient movement artifacts may be present.[19–23] The development of spinal phased array coils and fast sequences with flow compensation has enabled rapid imaging of the entire spinal cord within a reasonable time.[24] A large rectangular field of view of 48 cm (18.90 in) enables visualization of the entire spinal cord within one sagittal image. Motion suppression for heartbeats, lung movement, and swallowing using cardiac gating, saturation bands, and phase encoding in the head-feet direction further optimizes spinal cord MRI.[25]

SAGITTAL IMAGING

The gold standard MRI sequence to depict MS spinal cord abnormalities is dual-echo T2-weighted conventional spin echo (CSE), but other sequences, such as fast spin echo (FSE or TSE), short-tau inversion recovery (STIR), fluid attenuated inversion recovery (FLAIR), and gradient echo sequences also have been applied. Reports in literature are contradictory with regard to image quality and lesions sensitivity, with an exception for disappointing results using FLAIR sequences.[26–32]

Regardless of sequence of choice, dual echo T2-weighted MRI should be considered because it offers unique benefits with regard to artifact interpretation and lesion detection. With an appropriate first short TE, an intermediate-weighted image is obtained in which CSF appears isointense to the normal spinal cord. Consequently, high signal intensity of CSF and pulsation artifacts, as observed on more heavily T2-weighted images, no longer hinders image interpretation. Subtle MS abnormalities in the spinal cord, which are slightly hyperintense to CSF on intermediate-weighted image scan, can be depicted. For the detection of diffuse MS abnormalities in the spinal cord, an intermediate-weighted image is of critical value because the abnormalities may be easily missed on more heavily T2-weighted images. For lesion location within the cord, the second (T2) echo is also helpful (**Fig. 1**). Because of shorter acquisition time, FSE/TSE is preferred over CSE by some authors;[28,33,34] however, FSE has a possible lower sensitivity for spinal cord abnormalities, especially diffuse.

Reports that compared CSE and FSE/TSE sequences described nearly equal sensitivity for focal MS lesions in spinal cord (**Fig. 2**).[26,30] The use of a heavily T2-weighted single echo sequence alone decreased sensitivity for MS lesion detection substantially, however.[26,27] With regard to inversion recovery sequences, FLAIR is considered not suitable for spinal cord MRI,[26,28,29,35] although STIR or fast-STIR sequences seem to be useful for sagittal imaging and may depict additional lesions compared with CSE, although they are more susceptible to artifacts and less suitable as a stand-alone sequence.[31,36]

In contrast to brain MRI findings, MS abnormalities are only rarely seen on sagittal T1-weighted images. When hypointense lesions are observed in a differential diagnostic setting, other diseases, such as Devic's neuromyelitis optica (NMO) or even tumor, should be considered or excluded.[37] Enhancing lesions may be seen on T1-weighted images, representing active MS pathology (**Fig. 3**), although prevalence of these enhancing lesions is low compared with that of the brain.[34,38,39] In an imaging protocol, in addition to brain examination, acquiring only postcontrast T1-weighted images may suffice.

Axial Imaging

Axial imaging of the spinal cord is more difficult compared with sagittal imaging because of CSF pulsation and motion artifacts, which may hinder image quality, and the small cross-sectional size of the spinal cord. Axial imaging is less time efficient for the detection of cord MS abnormalities because of structure geometry. Sagittal imaging is usually preferred, although axial imaging may serve as confirmation of MR findings on sagittal images. In the axial plane, high-resolution sequences are needed because of the small cross-sectional areas of lesions and spinal cord. Slice thickness of 3 to 4 mm and a pixel size of 1 mm^2 or less are preferred to obtain enough anatomic information, such as the location of abnormalities in specific columns and relation to central gray matter, besides contrast to noise of lesions compared with normal-appearing white matter (NAWM). Within the spinal cord, the different anatomy of the venous anastomosing network, compared with the brain, causes MS lesions to be primarily wedge shaped on axial sections[40,41] and mostly located in the lateral and posterior columns, although they may appear in any column or gray matter.[42–45]

Because of faster acquisition times and lower sensitivity to motion artifacts, TSE and gradient echo are usually preferred in the axial plane above

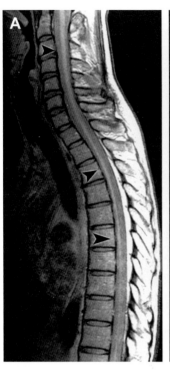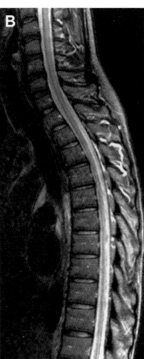

Fig. 1. Sagittal intermediate (*A*) and T2-weighted (*B*) dual echo spin echo images of the spinal cord. Note the diffuse abnormalities throughout the entire spinal cord as detected on the intermediate-weighted images. These abnormalities are difficult to appreciate on the T2-weighted image because of the high signal of CSF.

CSE. The quality of gradient echo images can be improved further by the application of a magnetization transfer (MT) presaturation pulse. Thin-slice, T2-weighted, three-dimensional, FSE/TSE sequences also increase the detection of MS lesions[46] but are more time consuming and artifact prone than two-dimensional FSE/TSE sequences. Comparison of sagittal and axial imaging for detection of MS abnormalities has not yet been studied, and no data have been published with regard to detection of diffuse abnormalities or differentiation of these abnormalities from focal lesions in the axial plane.

Depending on level of imaging, the size of the spinal cord may range from approximately 50 mm^2 to 100 mm^2. In healthy controls, 90 mm^2 at level C2 may be considered normal; however, a large variability in size has been described,[47–49] which limits the use for comparison of individuals. For measurement of the cross-sectional cord area (or volume), a heavily T1-weighted three-dimensional data set can be used to image voxels of approximately 1 mm^3.

Diffuse and Focal Spinal Cord Abnormalities

MS spinal cord abnormalities consist of two types: focal lesions and diffuse abnormalities.[30,39,50–55] Focal lesions are usually approximately one vertebra (maximum two segments) in length, are sharply delineated, are oval-shaped on the sagittal image, and are seen equally well on intermediate- and T2-weighted MRI.[56] The so-called diffuse abnormalities are typically observed on intermediate-weighted MRI as areas of increased signal intensity, which is higher compared with that of the surrounding CSF (see **Fig. 1**).[7] This diffuse abnormal signal is not well demarcated and is usually several segments long, although it appears frequently up to the whole length of the spinal cord and can be present in the entire diameter. Such diffuse abnormalities are difficult to recognize on T2-weighted images because spinal cord signal intensity is still lower than surrounding CSF.[7,26]

On dual-echo SE images, focal spinal cord abnormalities in MS are often multiple. In a cohort of patients who were recently diagnosed with MS, already more than a median of three focal lesions were described,[39] although a large range of abnormalities may be found, varying from a single focal lesion to a diffusely involved spinal cord with cases showing both focal and diffuse abnormalities (**Fig. 4**). The latter is mostly the case in patients who have more advanced MS.[57] Slightly more than 50% of focal cord lesions are found in the cervical cord. In the axial plane, these lesions are typically seen in the lateral and posterior columns and do not spare the central gray matter (**Fig. 5**).[56,58] They rarely cause focal swelling or atrophy of the spinal cord.[39] In cases of more advanced MS, focal

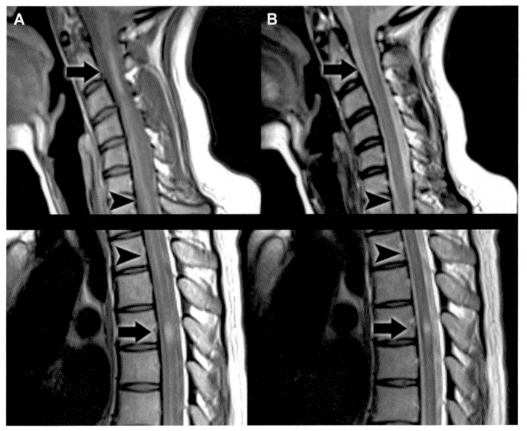

Fig. 2. Sagittal intermediate (*A*) and T2-weighted (*B*) dual echo FSE images of the spinal cord. Note the presence of both focal (*arrows*) and diffuse abnormalities (*arrowheads*). The diffuse abnormalities are more easily appreciated on the intermediate-weighted images. Also note the effect of long echo time on the appearance of the cervical focal lesion.

lesions may merge and form large confluent areas of high signal intensity exceeding two segments in length.[7] Some patients may only show diffuse abnormalities along the entire cord length.[7,59]

PREVALENCE OF SPINAL CORD ABNORMALITIES AND RELATION TO THE MULTIPLE SCLEROSIS CLINICAL PHENOTYPE

Prevalence of cord abnormalities in established MS is high, even in early stages of the disease. When focal and diffuse abnormalities are combined, up to 97% of patients who have MS may have abnormal spinal cord examinations.[7,59] Results in publications may vary depending on patient selection and the imaging method used. In clinically isolated syndromes, the prevalence of spinal cord lesions is lower,[60] especially if no spinal cord symptoms are present. Asymptomatic cord lesions are found in 30% to 40% of patients with clinically isolated syndromes, however;[61,62] according to Poser, in patients who have recently

diagnosed MS, criteria prevalence of abnormal cord examination may increase up to 83%.[39]

With regard to the type and the extent of spinal cord abnormalities and MS phenotypes, a trend has been described.[7] In patients who have relapsing-remitting MS (RRMS), spinal cord lesions typically consist of multiple focal lesions. In secondary progressive MS, abnormalities are more extensive; besides focal lesions, diffuse abnormalities are seen more frequently than in patients who have RRMS. Focal lesions also may become confluent as large, sharply delineated areas of high signal intensity. Spinal cord atrophy is common in this stage of the disease.[59] In patients who have primary progressive MS (PPMS), cord abnormalities are extensive compared with brain abnormalities.[33] In patients who have PPMS, focal and diffuse abnormalities have been described, although compared with the other MS phenotypes, diffuse abnormalities are more frequent.[7,59] Imaging the spinal cord may help to diagnose PPMS in patients with few or no brain abnormalities.

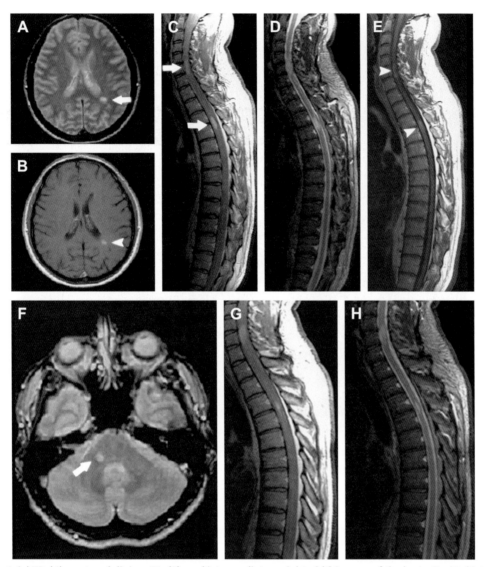

Fig. 3. Axial T2- (*A*), post-gadolinium T1- (*B*), and intermediate-weighted (*F*) images of the brain. Sagittal interme-diate- (*C, G*) and T2-weighted (*D, H*) dual echo spin echo images of the spinal cord are shown. Images A to E were obtained at first examination of a patient with a clinically isolated syndrome suggestive of MS showing one focal periventricular lesion (*arrow*) that enhanced after gadolinium (*arrowhead*). Initial brain examination showed no other brain lesions. Sagittal intermediate- (*C*) and T2-weighted (*D*) spinal cord images show two focal lesions (*ar-rows*) that both enhanced (*E, arrowheads*). Within differential diagnostics, acute disseminated encephalomyelitis was considered because all detected T2 lesions were enhancing. Criteria for dissemination in time or place were not met. Follow-up examination after 3 months, without clinical signs of relapse, showed a new infratentorial lesion (*F, arrow*) that did not enhance. No new focal spinal cord lesions or enhancement was observed in spinal cord examination. Oligoclonal bands were detected in CSF, and the patient was diagnosed with MS.

USE OF GADOLINIUM

To appreciate disease activity and new lesion for-mation in a single MR examination, one has to ac-quire T1-weighted imaging after intravenous injection of gadolinium (Gd) in addition to T2-weighted imaging.[63] Enhancing MS lesions on T1-weighted MRI after Gd injection reflect a disruption in the blood-brain barrier and active inflammation.[64,65] Because the degree of leakage depends on the time after injection, a postinjection delay of 15 to 30 minutes should be considered.

Although the value of adding Gd-enhanced T1-weighted imaging in spinal cord studies has not been assessed as thoroughly as in the brain, de-layed enhanced T1-weighted MRI may help to

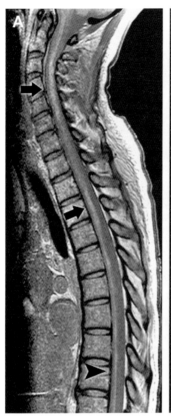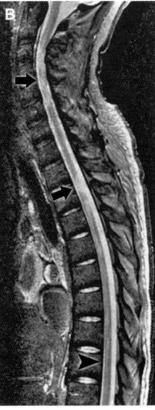

Fig. 4. Sagittal intermediate- (A) and T2-weighted (B) dual echo spin echo images of the spinal cord of a patient who had secondary progressive MS. Note the extensive abnormalities, both confluent focal (arrows) and diffuse at mid-thoracic level and in the caudal part of the spinal cord (arrowhead).

detect active spinal cord lesions in suspected cases of MS.[66] Enhancing lesions seem to be found much less frequently in the spinal cord than in the brain,[34,38] which limits the use of Gd enhancement in monitoring MS activity in the spinal cord. Enhancing MS cord lesions are usually small, no longer than two segments in cranial caudal length, are single, and show no or little

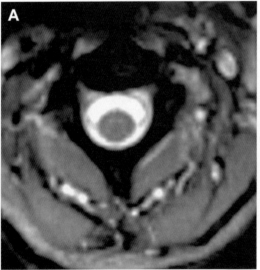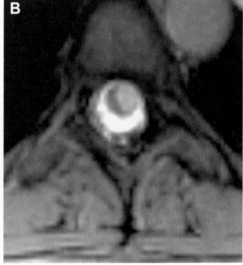

Fig. 5. Axial T2-weighted gradient echo images: normal cord (A) and spinal cord with a focal MS lesion (B). Note that the lesion does not spare the central gray matter and is located within the lateral, posterior, and anterior column on the left side. No focal swelling or atrophy of the cord is present.

perifocal edema or swelling of the cord. Gd enhancement in the spinal cord is often associated with new spinal cord symptoms (**Fig. 6**).[34] Adding postcontrast T1-weighted images to spinal cord MRI may be useful only when a new spinal cord lesion is suspected as the cause of a clinical relapse or when other diseases need to be excluded.

BRAIN AND SPINAL CORD ABNORMALITIES OCCUR INDEPENDENTLY

In cross-sectional studies, no clear relation between the number of spinal cord lesions and the number or location of brain lesions has been found, which indicates that spinal cord abnormalities occur largely independently of brain lesions.[33,39,59] No relation has been found between spinal cord atrophy and measurements of brain atrophy or number of brain lesions. To some extent, a relationship still seems plausible because brain abnormalities may cause secondary effects in the spinal cord, such as Wallerian degeneration.[34,67] A relationship was found between T1 relaxation time measurements of brain tissue and spinal cord.[68] Results also may be interpreted as an expression of diffuse disease involvement in brain and spinal cord, however.

THE CLINICORADIOLOGIC PARADOX: MRI CORRELATION WITH SYMPTOMS AND DISABILITY

A patient who has MS and little or no disability may have extensive brain MR abnormalities, whereas another patient with severe disability may have fewer abnormalities. This phenomenon is called the clinicoradiologic paradox.[69] Solving this paradox, besides improving early diagnosis, is probably the most important research goal of MR research in patients who have MS.

There may be several causes for the poor correlation between conventional MRI and disability (Expanded Disability Status Scale). Among these factors, one should consider the lack of spatial resolution[70] and, more importantly, the lack of pathologic specificity of T2-weighted MRI in MS.[71] T2-weighted spinal cord abnormalities and clinical findings are only weakly associated.[33,52,72,73] Compared with brain lesions, newly formed spinal cord lesions seem to be more related with new MS symptoms,[34,38] although clinically silent lesions do occur in patients who have MS.[53,54,73,74] Not all MS lesions in the spinal cord are clinically relevant. As in the brain, this may be caused by pathologic heterogeneity within spinal MS lesions.

To take a broad view: patients who have MS with spinal cord abnormalities are usually more disabled;[52] patients who have PPMS tend to have the most extensive involvement, patients who have secondary progressive MS have intermediate involvement, and patients who have RRMS have the smallest spinal cord involvement when considering focal lesions and diffuse abnormalities.[59] Diffuse cord abnormalities are associated with spinal symptoms, severe disability, and a PP disease course.[59]

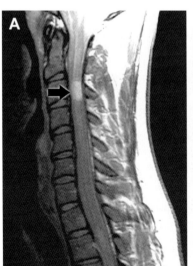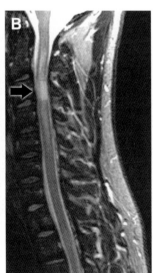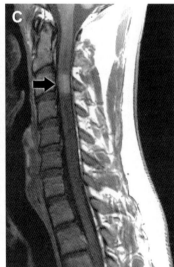

Fig. 6. Sagittal intermediate- (*A*) and T2-weighted (*B*) dual echo spin echo images and T1-weighted spin echo image after gadolinium injection (*C*) of the spinal cord in a patient who presented with clinical signs suggestive of acute partial transverse myelitis. Note the focal lesion (*arrow*) that is surrounded by edema (*B*), an uncommon finding in MS lesions, with little or no clear swelling of the cord. After administration of gadolinium (*C*), the lesion was clearly enhanced.

Currently, the best correlation between conventional MRI parameters and the Expanded Disability Status Scale has been found using spinal cord cross-sectional area/atrophy measurements.[48,75,76] Spinal cord atrophy seems to be more severe in patients who have PPMS and secondary progressive MS,[75] and it correlates with the appearance of diffuse abnormalities on sagittal MRI and disability.[59] Spinal cord atrophy may occur independently of the amount of focal cord lesions,[49] which suggests that the pathologic heterogeneity of spinal MS abnormalities exists and that mechanisms other than focal demyelination may be responsible for spinal cord atrophy.[77] The changes in cross-sectional area of spinal cord are small,[38,48,60,78] especially when compared with the wide range of cross-sectional area in healthy controls. As a consequence, the clinical use of spinal cord atrophy measurement is limited; however, there is a potential role for this measurement in long-term treatment trials aimed at the prevention of progressive tissue loss.[79]

The clinicoradiologic paradox indicates that pathologic changes are variable between MS lesions and also must be present outside focal MS abnormalities. To study MS lesions and NAWM changes objectively, new quantitative MR techniques must be considered and findings from this approach must be assessed in terms of their histopathologic substrate.

HISTOPATHOLOGIC ASSOCIATIONS

Only a few postmortem studies that have compared histopathologic changes in the spinal cord with MR characteristics in patients who have MS have been performed.[42,44,57] A strong correlation between the extent of demyelination and signal intensity abnormalities, as depicted with high-resolution, intermediate-weighted MR images, was described. Signal intensity increases on intermediate-weighted images were not specific for axonal loss, however. Histopathologic findings described were heterogeneous and ranged from demyelination with active inflammation to severe gliosis. Axonal loss seemed to occur independently of demyelination and was described in focal and diffuse signal intensity abnormalities and was extensively present in the NAWM. Up to 30% of axonal loss in NAWM of spinal cords of patients who have MS compared with white matter of control individuals was found—a pathologic condition that was not visible on intermediate-weighted images at 4.7 T. Whether this finding is the result of Wallerian degeneration, a diffuse axonal injury process, or both remains unclear.

Quantitative MR techniques have revealed differences in relaxation times and magnetization exchange properties between controls and MS cases; quantitative MRI also revealed differences between types of MS histopathology.[44] The degree of MR abnormality was found to be dominated by demyelination rather than axonal pathology, however. In contrast to the brain, T1 relaxation times were not able to distinguish between white matter of control specimens and NAWM. This phenomenon is apparently different from the situation in brain tissue, in which axonal loss is accompanied not only by atrophy but also by widening of extracellular spaces, which leads to abnormal relaxation mechanisms that are expressed on T1-weighted brain images as "black holes."[69,80] These differences may be explained by the central location of gray matter in the spinal cord, in contrast to brain, and consequently by the possibility of white matter collapse and resulting atrophy of the cord.

With regard to spinal cord atrophy, good correlations have been described with T1 relaxation time increase (and to a lesser extent with MT ratio [MTR] decrease and T2 relaxation time increase). Because these MR parameters are likely to primarily represent demyelination, it seems that cord atrophy itself is a feature that represents not only axonal loss but also loss of myelin, in which axonal density variance may occur independently of myelin density. This finding suggests that cord area measurement, which has been proposed as a clinically relevant marker for disease progression,[34,59,76,81] may not be regarded as a direct measure of the number of axons present in the spinal cord.[44] Considering initial promising results with regard to relation of clinical disability scores and diffusion-weighted (DW) MRI, it would be of interest to perform high-resolution DW MRI and relate findings with quantitative histopathology to define DW MRI sensitivity to axonal loss and demyelination.

DIFFERENTIAL DIAGNOSIS

In a diagnostic setting, spinal cord MRI seems to play a major role when differentiating MS from other CNS disease if used in addition to brain MRI.[55,82] Differential diagnostic considerations and consequent imaging planning first should take into account clinical presentation:[83] whether a patient presents with a first or new symptom in addition to old or previous symptoms. Second, it is important to realize whether the patient presents with spinal cord symptoms and whether the lesions found on MRI (if any) are perhaps clinically silent. Spinal cord MRI may be performed to detect MS abnormalities or rule out other diseases in case of normal or equivocal brain MRI (Fig. 7).

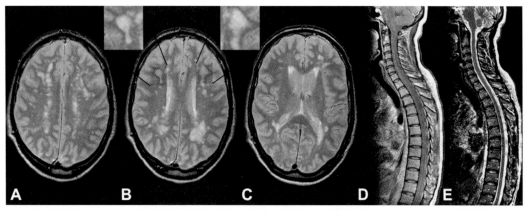

Fig. 7. Axial intermediate-weighted images of the brain (*A–C*) and intermediate- (*D*) and T2-weighted (*E*) dual echo spin echo images of the spinal cord from a patient with cerebrovascular disease. Brain images clearly show multiple focal white matter lesions, partially periventricularly and in the corpus callosum. Also note that lesions are spared the cortical u-fibers (see detail of image in *B*), a typical finding in vascular lesions. Images of the spinal cord were normal.

The differential diagnosis of focal high-signal-intensity lesions in the spinal cord includes vascular disorders, infectious disease, metabolic disorders (eg, vitamin B_{12} deficiency), radiation, neoplasm (eg, metastasis, astrocytoma), systemic disorders (eg, systemic lupus erythematosus, sarcoidosis), and degenerative, compressive, and traumatic conditions. Many of these disorders may also mimic MS on brain MRI scans, most importantly ischemic cerebrovascular diseases in elderly patients and patients with hypertension. In contrast to the brain, however, incidental (vascular) lesions rarely occur in the spinal cord,[1] even in patients with vascular brain pathologic conditions or cerebrovascular risk factors.[55] In contrast to MS, prevalence of incidental spinal cord lesions in other diseases seems low to almost nonexistent.

Outside of clinical presentations with a spinal cord syndrome, MRI of the spinal cord may be considered a powerful tool to differentiate MS from these other CNS conditions when brain MRI results are negative or equivocal.[55] A negative/normal spinal cord examination result may help to rule out MS in such cases. In case of a spinal cord syndrome or transverse myelitis, extent of the lesions in sagittal and axial planes enhancement pattern and clinical presentation should be assessed carefully in the diagnostic evaluation.[84–86] Lesion characteristics more typical of MS are as follows: preferably multifocal with combination of enhancing and nonenhancing lesions, lesions no longer than two vertebral segments in length, lesions that usually partially extend into the axial plane, and clinical presentation of partial transverse myelitis without back

pain or leptomeningeal enhancement. Local edema or swelling of the spinal cord may be present, although it is usually less extensive compared with other diseases that present with a transverse myelitis. Recurrence of partial transverse myelitis, without persisting T1 abnormalities, favors the diagnosis of MS.

ACUTE INFLAMMATORY DEMYELINATING DISORDERS OF THE SPINAL CORD

In addition to MS, inflammatory demyelinating disorders include Devic's NMO, acute transverse myelitis, and acute disseminated encephalomyelitis.[11,84,87–98]

Neuromyelitis Optica

In the "pure" form of NMO, MR abnormalities are typically restricted to the optic nerve and spinal cord (**Fig. 8**). In the acute phase, spinal cord abnormalities are typically large and show an extensive, inhomogeneous enhancement and swelling of the cord. In the chronic phase, enhancement fades away and focal atrophy in combination with T1 hypointense abnormalities (cystic changes) may become visible. In cases of NMO, however, abnormalities elsewhere in the CNS may be present and delay the correct diagnosis. Within a diagnostic setting, presence of AQP4 autoantibodies, NMO-IGg, in CSF may differentiate NMO from MS. In contrast, MS lesions tend to exhibit stage-dependent loss of AQP4.[99–103]

Acute Transverse Myelitis

Imaging characteristics of a spinal cord lesion in acute transverse myelitis are defined by a large,

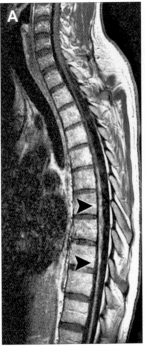
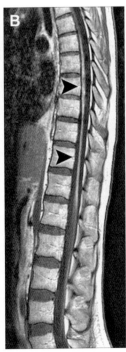
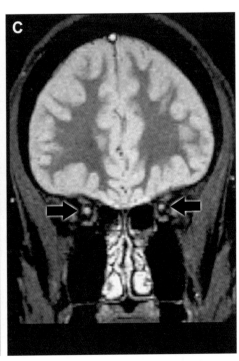

Fig. 8. Sagittal T1-weighted spin echo images of the spinal cord (*A, B*), coronal fast STIR of the optic nerve of a patient with Devic's NMO. Spinal cord images show extensive, multisegmental, inhomogeneously enhancing abnormalities (*arrowheads*) in combination with (*C*) bilateral optic neuritis (arrows) in the absence of any brain lesion. The right optic nerve appears more swollen.

multisegmental focal lesion that is more than two vertebrae in length and usually shows swelling, edema, and extensive enhancement in the acute phase. Imaging characteristics and clinical presentation may differentiate from MS. In case of similar imaging and clinical characteristics, differential diagnosis should consider anterior spinal artery thrombosis, dural arteriovenous fistula, MS, and NMO. A diagnosis of acute transverse myelitis also should be excluded after the diagnostic guidelines for acute transverse myelitis are consulted (**Fig. 9**).[86]

Acute Disseminated Encephalomyelitis

With a monophasic appearance that typically shows multiple enhancing lesions in brain or spinal cord, acute disseminated encephalomyelitis initially may be difficult to differentiate from clinically isolated syndrome suggestive of MS. Most cases are seen in childhood, however, commonly within a short interval after a viral infection.[104] Suggestive features of acute disseminated encephalomyelitis include multiple simultaneously enhancing T2 lesions in the brain and spinal cord, more extensive cord involvement, and more edematous changes than MS. Clinical and MRI follow-up is important to rule out dissemination in space and time that favors the diagnosis of (childhood) MS.

Other Inflammatory Diseases

In contrast to the brain, MS-like abnormalities are seldom found in the spinal cord of patients with OIDs such as sarcoidosis and systemic lupus erythematosus. When present, such abnormalities may differ from those seen in cases of MS.[8–18] Spinal cord lesions in OID are generally symptomatic, which is not often seen in cases of MS, in which asymptomatic spinal cord lesions are common. One study reported no focal cervical cord lesions in 44 patients who had OID,[82] although 30% showed brain abnormalities that mimicked MS.[105] In sarcoidosis and systemic lupus erythematosus, the use of Gd may reveal leptomeningeal involvement, a feature rarely seen in MS. In these disorders, spinal cord abnormalities consist of diffuse signal changes and, in some cases, focal changes. These abnormalities are probably secondary to the leptomeningeal involvement.

DIAGNOSTIC CRITERIA FOR MRI IN MULTIPLE SCLEROSIS: SPINAL CORD MRI IN THE DIAGNOSTIC SETTING

Classically, the most important diagnostic principle for MS disease is the presence of dissemination in space and time. Clinical and MRI findings are critical for the diagnosis of MS as formulated

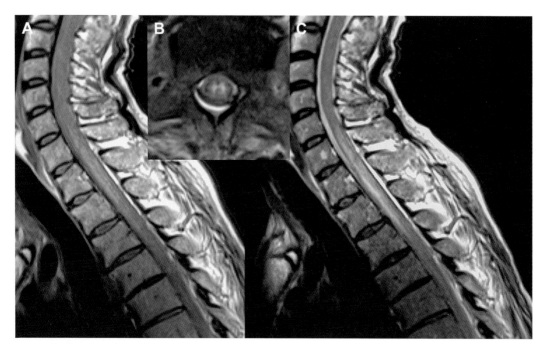

Fig. 9. Sagittal intermediate- (*A*) and T2-weighted (*C*) dual echo spin echo images. (*B*) Axial T2-weighted gradient echo image. Images were obtained from a patient with an acute spinal cord syndrome caused by an anterior spinal artery infarct. The intermediate- and T2-weighted images show an inhomogeneous multisegmental area of edema around moderately swollen and strongly hyperintense central gray matter caused by cytotoxic edema.

by McDonald.[83,106] MRI has become the method of choice for obtaining evidence of dissemination in space and time as a paraclinical confirmation of the clinical diagnosis.[107] The demonstration of multiple T2 lesions in characteristic locations suggests dissemination in space. The presence of nonenhancing and Gd-enhancing lesions is suggestive of dissemination in time.

MRI Criteria for Relapse-Onset Multiple Sclerosis

To increase MR specificity for MS, diagnostic criteria were developed based on the number, location, size, and enhancement of brain lesions.[3–5] With increasing specificity, the sensitivity of the criteria reduces as a result of an increased number of lesions at specific locations necessary to fulfill the criteria. To increase sensitivity, Tintore and colleagues[108] modified the Barkhof criteria[5] for dissemination in space. Of the four conditions formulated by Barkhof and colleagues, three have to be fulfilled.[83] In examinations without Gd enhancement, nine T2 lesions may substitute for the presence of an enhancing lesion. Substitution of brain lesions by spinal cord abnormalities to meet the Barkhof/Tintore criteria was introduced by the McDonald panel and later revised by Polman and colleagues.[106]

Within the original McDonald criteria, the interpretation of the "substitution rule" for cord lesions was unclear and revised in the most recent version of this diagnostic classification. A focal spinal cord lesion is equivalent to and may substitute for an infratentorial lesion but not for a periventricular or a juxtacortical lesion. An enhancing spinal cord lesion is equivalent to an enhancing brain lesion, and an enhancing spinal cord lesion can count for an enhancing lesion and an infratentorial lesion. Individual spinal cord lesions can contribute together with individual brain lesions to reach the required nine T2 lesions. Diffuse abnormalities were considered not sufficiently reliable and explicitly not included within the criteria.

Diagnostic Criteria for Primary Progressive Multiple Sclerosis

The revised McDonald criteria for PPMS place more emphasis on spinal cord MRI because few brain lesions are commonly detected in this patient group. For these criteria, a patient who has PPMS should be observed over a period of 1 year and show signs of gradual disease progression and a combination of at least two of the following items: nine T2 lesions or four T2 lesions and positive visual evoked potentials, two focal spinal cord lesions, and IgG oligoclonal banding in the CSF. As formulated in the original and revised McDonald criteria, eliminating any other neurologic disorder that might explain the clinical and MRI findings in a patient is mandatory before a diagnosis of MS is considered. Because spinal cord symptoms are frequent in patients who have PPMS, any disease that may cause cord symptoms, such as dural arteriovenous fistula or compressive spinal cord disease, needs to be excluded. To expand the concept of "no better explanation," Charil and colleagues[109] defined a series of MRI red flags that pointed in a direction other than MS in the clinical setting of suspected MS. The role of spinal cord MRI is especially important in the diagnosis of PPMS, which often presents with spinal cord symptoms only.

INDICATIONS FOR SPINAL CORD MRI AT DIAGNOSIS AND FOLLOW-UP EXAMINATION

Each patient with possible MS should undergo brain MRI (**Table 1**). If the results are unequivocal and there is no clinical evidence of spinal cord involvement, spinal cord MRI is not needed. On the contrary, spinal cord MRI is needed when results of brain MRI are inconclusive (negative with high clinical suspicion or possibly associated with a vascular disease), when spinal cord involvement is suspected clinically, or when patients have a progressive-onset presentation. In patients in whom the criteria of dissemination in space or time—necessities for the clinical diagnosis of MS—have not been fulfilled, serial MRI can be used to demonstrate new lesions at follow-up. The interval to detect new T2 lesions, as defined in recently revised McDonald criteria,[106] was set at 30 days. For a new enhancing T1 lesion, the interval was defined as 3 months.

Serial spinal cord MRI in addition to brain MRI is not routinely indicated. Incidence of newly formed or enhancing spinal cord lesions is low compared with that of brain lesions, especially when no new cord symptoms are present. Proposed MRI protocol for patients suspected of having MS or follow-up examination can be found in **Box 1**.

FUTURE DEVELOPMENTS: NEW MRI TECHNIQUES

T2-weighted MRI, in vivo at 1.5 T, has suboptimal sensitivity, specificity, and spatial resolution to depict MS pathology in the spinal cord. To increase detection of pathologic state, an increase of field strength—and consequently spatial resolution—may increase sensitivity for smaller lesions. Nonconventional quantitative MRI techniques also should be explored, however, to increase the sensitivity to detect, quantify, and define the nature of abnormalities such as demyelination and axonal loss in NAWM and T2-visible lesions. With new generation MRI scanners, these technically challenging MR techniques may become feasible for clinical applications. To date, however, these techniques are difficult to perform, especially in the spinal cord. With increasing complex and quantitative techniques, the effects of magnetic field, coil, and pulse inhomogeneities (besides challenges with spatial resolution, susceptibility artifacts and macroscopic motion) become factors increasingly difficult but important to cope with. More studies have to be performed to verify histopathologic specificity for these new quantitative techniques. The following section discusses the most promising quantitative MRI techniques.

Magnetization Transfer MRI

By obtaining two images, one with and one without an off-resonance presaturation pulse, MTR maps can be calculated. Using this technique, information may be obtained with regard to the

Table 1 Indications for spinal cord imaging	
Situation	**Goal**
Clinically isolated syndrome with only spinal cord symptoms	Increase specificity and sensitivity, rule out other disease, or detect clinically silent lesions
Negative brain scan and strong clinical suspicion	Increase sensitivity, detect additional MS lesions
Nonspecific brain MRI findings (eg, older age, hypertension)	Increase specificity, determine whether absence of spinal cord lesions may rule out MS
Atypical new spinal cord symptoms	Increase specificity, rule out other disease, or confirm MS lesions
Primary progressive MS	Increase sensitivity and specificity, detect additional lesions (or diffuse abnormalities), rule out other disease

In case of conclusive brain MR examination and no clinical evidence for spinal cord involvement, there are no indications for additional spinal cord imaging.

Box 1
Proposed imaging protocol for McDonald criteria (1.5 T)

Brain MR

    Circularly polarized head coil

    Axial pregadolinium axial T1-weighted CSE (eg, 630/14/2[TR/TE/excitations])

    Sagittal turbo-FLAIR (eg, 9000/2500/108/1 [TR/Ti/TE/excitations])

    Gadolinium injection, 0.3 mmol/kg

    Axial dual-echo long TR CSE images (eg, 2700/45;90/1)

    Axial postgadolinium axial T1-weighted CSE (eg, 630/14/2)

(48 slices, 3-mm slice thickness, 0.3-mm inter-slice gap, 172 × 250 mm field of view and a 176 × 256 matrix).

Spinal MR

    Spinal phased array coil

    Sagittal postgadolinium T1-weighted TSE (729/14/2)

    Sagittal long TR dual-echo TSE (3000/15;117/1)

(13 slices, 3-mm slice thickness, 0.3-mm inter-slice gap, 240 × 480 mm field of view and 256 × 512 matrix).

---

amount of macromolecules present in the acquired volume, such as myelin, and may provide quantitative data about the integrity of CNS parenchyma. Relative MTR decreases in the brain relate to the degree of tissue destruction[71] and clinical findings.[110,111] In the brain and spinal cord, MTRs are lower in MS lesions and NAWM compared with normal white matter of healthy controls.[112] In a study based on histogram analysis, no difference was found between control subjects and patients with RRMS, whereas patients who had PPMS and secondary progressive MS had abnormal MTR histogram results. Cervical cord histogram measures were independent predictors of locomotor disability.[113] As described in a postmortem spinal cord study, MTR decrease was found to relate mostly to presence of myelin/demyelination,[44] and no independent relation between MTR and axonal densities could be found.

Diffusion-Weighted MRI

Currently, a technically challenging but feasible and promising technique for detection and estimation of spinal cord damage is DW MRI and diffusion tensor MRI.[113] Recent studies using this technique have shown the possibility of achieving an accurate estimation of the extent of cervical cord damage in MS and other diseases of the spinal cord.[114–117] Some studies have described a good correlation between changes in fractional anisotropy and mean diffusivity and markers for clinical disability in cross-sectional studies (r values ranging from 0.36–0.58).[115,118] In a follow-up study, baseline cord cross-sectional area (r = −0.40, P = .01) and fractional anisotropy (r = −0.40, P = .03) correlated with increase in disability at follow-up.[118] In patients who have MS, decrease in cord cross-sectional area and fractional anisotropy and increase in cervical cord mean diffusivity have been described compared with healthy controls and between MS phenotypes. Between patients who have PPMS and patients who have other MS phenotypes, cord fractional anisotropy decrease was found but not mean diffusivity or cord cross-sectional area measurement differences.[114,118]

No clear relation could be found between brain and cord metrics, and mean diffusivity and fractional anisotropy showed independent contribution to disability in a multivariate linear regression model with a correlation coefficient of 0.73 (P < .001).[115] Data from these studies may indicate that spinal cord changes are not merely dependent of changes in the brain and that pathologic evolution may develop at different rates in different patients. Histopathologic changes within the cord may be twofold: tissue loss and injury to remaining tissue may be two separate components that are not strictly interrelated, which was a finding previously suggested with regard to the relation of cord atrophy, axonal loss, and relaxation time measurements. MS cord pathology also seemed to develop at different rates according to disease phenotype and was associated with an increase in disability.

Proton Magnetic Resonance Spectroscopy

Assessment of N-acetyl aspartate (NAA) with proton MR spectroscopy (^{1}H-MRS) is one of the most specific measures of axonal damage in the brain and spinal cord,[119] because NAA is almost exclusively contained in neurons and axons. In recent studies, feasibility of ^{1}H-MRS in spinal cord has been shown and compared with brain and clinical findings.[120–123] Reduction of NAA was detected in spinal cord (32% decrease, $P < .05$), whereas NAA in the brain was not significantly altered. No correlation between clinical measures and cord atrophy or brain lesion volume was found; however, spinal cord NAA correlated with the cerebellar subscore of the neurologic assessment ($P < .005$). ^{1}H-MRS demonstrated cellular damage within the cord over and above the tissue atrophy seen with conventional MRI. Combining MRI and ^{1}H-MRS may give a more complete picture of neurodegeneration in the spinal cord. Another study that described relation of other detected metabolites with the Expanded Disability Status Scale and DW/diffusion tensor MRI parameters concluded that ^{1}H-MRS and diffusion-based tractography of the cervical cord can provide measures that are sensitive to tissue damage occurring in this area in patients with a cervical cord relapse.[124] These measures were found to correlate with acute disability, and longitudinal studies should be performed and extended to other neurologic diseases that affect the spinal cord.[124]

Functional MRI

Possibly the most technically challenging MRI technique for spinal cord imaging, functional MRI has become feasible and reliable. Using peripheral cardiac pulsation registration to correct for motion induced errors, blood oxygen level–dependent signal changes can de detected within the spinal cord gray matter during different passive motor or sensory paradigms.[125–132] Functional MRI already has detected differences between patients who have MS and healthy controls, with a general pattern of recruitment and increased blood oxygen level–dependent signal intensity changes in patients who have MS.[133] In another study, patients who had RRMS showed abnormal recruitment patterns compared with controls during passive motor and sensory tasks.[134] During paradigms of thermal stimulation, the patients who had RRMS showed similar activation patterns compared with controls, whereas patients who had PPMS

showed a recruitment pattern similar to patients with spinal cord trauma. A future role of functional MRI of the spinal cord will most likely be the cornerstone of understanding the adaptive role and detecting definite irreversible damage within the spinal cord and estimating disease progression.

SUMMARY

MS is a diffuse disease of the CNS, and MRI of the spinal cord is highly recommended in the clinical evaluation of patients suspected of having MS. With current conventional MRI techniques, spinal cord MRI of sufficient resolution within reasonable time is feasible for diagnostic purposes. Current clinically applicable MRI techniques should be considered reasonably sensitive to detect demyelination, although they are neither specific nor sensitive enough to detect axonal loss. Spinal cord MRI findings facilitate early diagnosis of MS in patients who have clinically isolated syndromes. When used with brain findings, the increase in sensitivity of MRI criteria for MS might not influence specificity because of the high prevalence of clinically silent cord lesions in patients who have MS compared with other CNS diseases. In the case of spinal cord symptoms, other diseases may be ruled out (and MS might be confirmed). Because the incidence of new spinal cord lesions without new cord symptoms clinically is low compared with brain, routine examination of the spinal cord is not indicated in the follow-up of patients who have MS.

Within the new diagnostic criteria, spinal cord MRI increases sensitivity and possibly specificity for MS, but further work is needed to investigate other criteria that may give greater weight to the presence of cord lesions in patients with clinically isolated syndromes or suspected RRMS to facilitate early diagnosis. With new technically complex quantitative MRI techniques, an increase in sensitivity for detection and specification of pathologic substrate may become feasible. Techniques should be further studied and validated in studies comparing these techniques with clinical status and histopathology, however.

REFERENCES

1. Thorpe JW, Kidd D, Kendall BE, et al. Spinal cord MRI using multi-array coils and fast spin echo. I. Technical aspects and findings in healthy adults. Neurology 1993;43:2625–31.
2. Solomon MA. MRI in MS diagnosis. Neurology 1987;37:1566–7.
3. Fazekas F, Offenbacher H, Fuchs S, et al. Criteria for an increased specificity of MRI interpretation

in elderly subjects with suspected multiple sclerosis. Neurology 1988;38:1822–5.

4. Paty DW, Oger JJ, Kastrukoff LF, et al. MRI in the diagnosis of MS: a prospective study with comparison of clinical evaluation, evoked potentials, oligoclonal banding, and CT. Neurology 1988;38:180–5.

5. Barkhof F, Filippi M, Miller DH, et al. Comparison of MRI criteria at first presentation to predict conversion to clinically definite multiple sclerosis. Brain 1997;120:2059–69.

6. Lee KH, Hashimoto SA, Hooge JP, et al. Magnetic resonance imaging of the head in the diagnosis of multiple sclerosis: a prospective 2-year follow-up with comparison of clinical evaluation, evoked potentials, oligoclonal banding, and CT. Neurology 1991;41:657–60.

7. Lycklama à Nijeholt GJ, Barkhof F, Scheltens P, et al. MR of the spinal cord in multiple sclerosis: relation to clinical subtype and disability. AJNR Am J Neuroradiol 1997;18:1041–8.

8. Provenzale JM, Barboriak DP, Gaensler EH, et al. Lupus-related myelitis: serial MR findings. AJNR Am J Neuroradiol 1994;15:1911–7.

9. Salmaggi A, Lamperti E, Eoli M, et al. Spinal cord involvement and systemic lupus erythematosus: clinical and magnetic resonance findings in 5 patients. Clin Exp Rheumatol 1994;12:389–94 [published erratum appears in Clin Exp Rheumatol 1994 Nov-Dec;12(6):695].

10. Simeon-Aznar CP, Tolosa-Vilella C, Cuenca-Luque R, et al. Transverse myelitis in systemic lupus erythematosus: two cases with magnetic resonance imaging. Br J Rheumatol 1992;31:555–8.

11. Boumpas DT, Patronas NJ, Dalakas MC, et al. Acute transverse myelitis in systemic lupus erythematosus: magnetic resonance imaging and review of the literature. J Rheumatol 1990;17:89–92.

12. Sobue G, Yasuda T, Kumazawa K, et al. MRI demonstrates dorsal column involvement of the spinal cord in Sjogren's syndrome-associated neuropathy. Neurology 1995;45:592–3.

13. Nishiura I, Tochio H, Koyama T. Cervical intramedullary sarcoidosis. Neurochirurgia (Stuttg) 1992;35:163–6.

14. Junger SS, Stern BJ, Levine SR, et al. Intramedullary spinal sarcoidosis: clinical and magnetic resonance imaging characteristics. Neurology 1993;43:333–7.

15. Lexa FJ, Grossman RI. MR of sarcoidosis in the head and spine: spectrum of manifestations and radiographic response to steroid therapy. AJNR Am J Neuroradiol 1994;15:973–82.

16. Nesbit GM, Miller GM, Baker HL Jr, et al. Spinal cord sarcoidosis: a new finding at MR imaging with Gd-DTPA enhancement. Radiology 1989;173:839–43.

17. Rieger J, Hosten N. Spinal cord sarcoidosis. Neuroradiology 1994;36:627–8.

18. Simon JH. The contribution of spinal cord MRI to the diagnosis and differential diagnosis of multiple sclerosis. J Neurol Sci 2000;172(Suppl 1):S32–5.

19. Bronskill MJ, McVeigh ER, Kucharczyk W, et al. Syrinx-like artifacts on MR images of the spinal cord. Radiology 1988;166:485–8.

20. Curtin AJ, Chakeres DW, Bulas R, et al. MR imaging artifacts of the axial internal anatomy of the cervical spinal cord. AJR Am J Roentgenol 1989;152:835–42.

21. Czervionke LF, Czervionke JM, Daniels DL, et al. Characteristic features of MR truncation artifacts. AJR Am J Roentgenol 1988;151:1219–28.

22. Hinks RS, Quencer RM. Motion artifacts in brain and spine MR. Radiol Clin North Am 1988;26:737–53.

23. Levy LM, Di CG, Brooks RA, et al. Spinal cord artifacts from truncation errors during MR imaging. Radiology 1988;166:479–83.

24. Roemer PB, Edelstein WA, Hayes CE, et al. The NMR phased array. Magn Reson Med 1990;16:192–225.

25. Mikulis DJ, Wood ML, Zerdoner OA, et al. Oscillatory motion of the normal cervical spinal cord. Radiology 1994;192:117–21.

26. Hittmair K, Mallek R, Prayer D, et al. Spinal cord lesions in patients with multiple sclerosis: comparison of MR pulse sequences. AJNR Am J Neuroradiol 1996;17:1555–65.

27. Bianco F. Is fast spin-echo superior to gradient-echo imaging in detecting spinal cord lesions or not? AJNR Am J Neuroradiol 1996;17:194 [letter].

28. Filippi M, Yousry TA, Alkadhi H, et al. Spinal cord MRI in multiple sclerosis with multicoil arrays: a comparison between fast spin echo and fast FLAIR. J Neurol Neurosurg Psychiatr 1996;61:632–5.

29. Stevenson VL, Gawne-Cain ML, Barker GJ, et al. Imaging of the spinal cord and brain in multiple sclerosis: a comparative study between fast FLAIR and fast spin echo. J Neurol 1997;244:119–24.

30. Lycklama à Nijeholt GJ, Castelijns JA, Weerts J, et al. Sagittal MR of multiple sclerosis in the spinal cord: fast versus conventional spin-echo imaging. Am J Neuroradiol 1998;19:355–60.

31. Bot JC, Barkhof F, Nijeholt GJ, et al. Comparison of a conventional cardiac-triggered dual spin-echo and a fast STIR sequence in detection of spinal cord lesions in multiple sclerosis. Eur Radiol 2000;10:753–8.

32. Sze G, Merriam M, Oshio K, et al. Fast spin-echo imaging in the evaluation of intradural disease of the spine. AJNR Am J Neuroradiol 1992;13:1383–92.

33. Kidd D, Thorpe JW, Thompson AJ, et al. Spinal cord MRI using multi-array coils and fast spin

echo. II. Findings in multiple sclerosis. Neurology 1993;43:2632–7.

34. Thorpe JW, Kidd D, Moseley IF, et al. Serial gadolinium-enhanced MRI of the brain and spinal cord in early relapsing-remitting multiple sclerosis. Neurology 1996;46:373–8.

35. Keiper MD, Grossman RI, Brunson JC, et al. The low sensitivity of fluid-attenuated inversion-recovery MR in the detection of multiple sclerosis of the spinal cord. AJNR Am J Neuroradiol 1997; 18:1035–9.

36. Dietemann JL, Thibaut-Menard A, Warter JM, et al. MRI in multiple sclerosis of the spinal cord: evaluation of fast short-tan inversion-recovery and spin-echo sequences. Neuroradiology 2000;42:810–3.

37. Cohen-Gadol AA, Zikel OM, Miller GM, et al. Spinal cord biopsy: a review of 38 cases. Neurosurgery 2003;52:806–15.

38. Kidd D, Thorpe JW, Kendall BE, et al. MRI dynamics of brain and spinal cord in progressive multiple sclerosis. J Neurol Neurosurg Psychiatr 1996;60: 15–9.

39. Bot JC, Barkhof F, Polman CH, et al. Spinal cord abnormalities in recently diagnosed MS patients: added value of spinal MRI examination. Neurology 2004;62:226–33.

40. Fog T. Topographic distribution of plaques in the spinal cord in multiple sclerosis. Arch Neurol Psychaiatry 1950;63:382–414.

41. Fog T. The topography of plaques in multiple sclerosis with special reference to cerebral plaques. Acta Neurol Scand, Suppl 1965;15:1–161.

42. Nijeholt GJ, Bergers E, Kamphorst W, et al. Postmortem high-resolution MRI of the spinal cord in multiple sclerosis: a correlative study with conventional MRI, histopathology and clinical phenotype. Brain 2001;124:154–66.

43. Bergers E, Bot JC, De Groot CJ, et al. Axonal damage in the spinal cord of MS patients occurs largely independent of T2 MRI lesions. Neurology 2002;59: 1766–71.

44. Bot JC, Blezer EL, Kamphorst W, et al. The spinal cord in multiple sclerosis: relationship of high-spatial-resolution quantitative MR imaging findings to histopathologic results. Radiology 2004;233: 531–40.

45. Filippi M, Rocca MA. MRI evidence for multiple sclerosis as a diffuse disease of the central nervous system. J Neurol 2005;252(Suppl 5):v16–24.

46. Stevenson VL, Moseley IF, Phatouros CC, et al. Improved imaging of the spinal cord in multiple sclerosis using three-dimensional fast spin echo. Neuroradiology 1998;40:416–9.

47. Kameyama T, Hashizume Y, Sobue G. Morphologic features of the normal human cadaveric spinal cord. Spine 1996;21:1285–90.

48. Stevenson VL, Leary SM, Losseff NA, et al. Spinal cord atrophy and disability in MS: a longitudinal study. Neurology 1998;51:234–8.

49. Evangelou N, DeLuca GC, Owens T, et al. Pathological study of spinal cord atrophy in multiple sclerosis suggests limited role of local lesions. Brain 2005;128:29–34.

50. Maravilla KR, Weinreb JC, Suss R, et al. Magnetic resonance demonstration of multiple sclerosis plaques in the cervical cord. AJR Am J Roentgenol 1985;144:381–5.

51. Edwards MK, Farlow MR, Stevens JC. Cranial MR in spinal cord MS: diagnosing patients with isolated spinal cord symptoms. AJNR Am J Neuroradiol 1986;7:1003–5.

52. Honig L, Sheremata W. Magnetic resonance imaging of spinal cord lesions in multiple sclerosis. J Neurol Neurosurg Psychiatr 1989;52:459–66.

53. Uldry PA, Regli F, Uske A. Magnetic resonance imaging in patients with multiple sclerosis and spinal cord involvement: 28 cases. J Neurol 1993;240:41–5.

54. Papadopoulos A, Gatzonis S, Gouliamos A, et al. Correlation between spinal cord MRI and clinical features in patients with demyelinating disease. Neuroradiology 1994;36:130–3.

55. Bot JC, Barkhof F, Nijeholt G, et al. Differentiation of multiple sclerosis from other inflammatory disorders and cerebrovascular disease: value of spinal MR imaging. Radiology 2002;223:46–56.

56. Tartaglino LM, Friedman DP, Flanders AE, et al. Multiple sclerosis in the spinal cord: MR appearance and correlation with clinical parameters. Radiology 1995;195:725–32.

57. Bergers E, Bot JC, van d V, et al. Diffuse signal abnormalities in the spinal cord in multiple sclerosis: direct postmortem in situ magnetic resonance imaging correlated with in vitro high-resolution magnetic resonance imaging and histopathology. Ann Neurol 2002;51:652–6.

58. Thielen KR, Miller GM. Multiple sclerosis of the spinal cord: magnetic resonance appearance. J Comput Assist Tomogr 1996;20:434–8.

59. Lycklama à Nijeholt GJ, Vanwalderveen MA, Castelijns JA, et al. Brain and spinal cord abnormalities in multiple sclerosis: correlation between MRI parameters, clinical subtypes and symptoms. Brain 1998;121:687–97.

60. Brex PA, Leary SM, O'Riordan JI, et al. Measurement of spinal cord area in clinically isolated syndromes suggestive of multiple sclerosis. J Neurol Neurosurg Psychiatr 2001;70:544–7.

61. O'Riordan JI, Losseff NA, Phatouros C, et al. Asymptomatic spinal cord lesions in clinically isolated optic nerve, brain stem, and spinal cord syndromes suggestive of demyelination. J Neurol Neurosurg Psychiatr 1998;64:353–7.

62. Brex PA, O'Riordan JI, Miszkiel KA, et al. Multisequence MRI in clinically isolated syndromes and the early development of MS. Neurology 1999;53: 1184–90.

63. Miller DH, Barkhof F, Nauta JJ. Gadolinium enhancement increases the sensitivity of MRI in detecting disease activity in multiple sclerosis. Brain 1993;116:1077–94.

64. Brasch RC, Weinmann HJ, Wesbey GE. Contrast-enhanced NMR imaging: animal studies using gadolinium-DTPA complex. AJR Am J Roentgenol 1984;142:625–30.

65. Carr DH, Gadian DG. Contrast agents in magnetic resonance imaging. Clin Radiol 1985;36:561–8.

66. Larsson EM, Holtas S, Nilsson O. Gd-DTPA-enhanced MR of suspected spinal multiple sclerosis. AJNR Am J Neuroradiol 1989;10:1071–6.

67. Silver NC, Good CD, Sormani MP, et al. A modified protocol to improve the detection of enhancing brain and spinal cord lesions in multiple sclerosis. J Neurol 2001;248:215–24.

68. Vaithianathar L, Tench CR, Morgan PS, et al. Magnetic resonance imaging of the cervical spinal cord in multiple sclerosis: a quantitative T1 relaxation time mapping approach. J Neurol 2003;250: 307–15.

69. Barkhof F, van Walderveen M. Characterization of tissue damage in multiple sclerosis by nuclear magnetic resonance. Philos Trans R Soc Lond, B, Biol Sci 1999;354:1675–86.

70. Bachmann R, Reilmann R, Schwindt W, et al. FLAIR imaging for multiple sclerosis: a comparative MR study at 1.5 and 3.0 Tesla. Eur Radiol 2006;16: 915–21.

71. van Waesberghe JH, Kamphorst W, De Groot CJ, et al. Axonal loss in multiple sclerosis lesions: magnetic resonance imaging insights into substrates of disability. Ann Neurol 1999;46:747–54.

72. Turano G, Jones SJ, Miller DH, et al. Correlation of SEP abnormalities with brain and cervical cord MRI in multiple sclerosis. Brain 1991;114:663–81.

73. Wiebe S, Lee DH, Karlik SJ, et al. Serial cranial and spinal cord magnetic resonance imaging in multiple sclerosis. Ann Neurol 1992;32:643–50.

74. Schneider U, Wullenweber M, Hrastnik K, et al. Nuclear magnetic resonance tomography in multiple sclerosis: comparison of spinal and cerebral findings. Nervenarzt 1995;66:129–32 [German].

75. Filippi M, Campi A, Colombo B, et al. A spinal cord MRI study of benign and secondary progressive multiple sclerosis. J Neurol 1996;243:502–5.

76. Losseff NA, Webb SL, O'Riordan JI, et al. Spinal cord atrophy and disability in multiple sclerosis: a new reproducible and sensitive MRI method with potential to monitor disease progression. Brain 1996;119:701–8.

77. Lin X, Tench CR, Evangelou N, et al. Measurement of spinal cord atrophy in multiple sclerosis. J Neuroimaging 2004;14:20S–6S.

78. Stevenson VL, Miller DH, Leary SM, et al. One year follow up study of primary and transitional progressive multiple sclerosis. J Neurol Neurosurg Psychiatr 2000;68:713–8.

79. Zivadinov R, Bakshi R. Role of MRI in multiple sclerosis II: brain and spinal cord atrophy. Front Biosci 2004;9:647–64.

80. van Walderveen MA, Barkhof F, Pouwels PJ, et al. Neuronal damage in T1-hypointense multiple sclerosis lesions demonstrated in vivo using proton magnetic resonance spectroscopy. Ann Neurol 1999;46:79–87.

81. Stevenson VL, Miller DH, Rovaris M, et al. Primary and transitional progressive MS: a clinical and MRI cross-sectional study. Neurology 1999;52: 839–45.

82. Rovaris M, Viti B, Ciboddo G, et al. Cervical cord magnetic resonance imaging findings in systemic immune-mediated diseases. J Neurol Sci 2000; 176:128–30.

83. McDonald WI, Compston A, Edan G, et al. Recommended diagnostic criteria for multiple sclerosis: guidelines from the international panel on the diagnosis of multiple sclerosis. Ann Neurol 2001;50: 121–7.

84. Jeffery DR, Mandler RN, Davis LE. Transverse myelitis: retrospective analysis of 33 cases, with differentiation of cases associated with multiple sclerosis and parainfectious events. Arch Neurol 1993;50:532–5.

85. de SJ, Stojkovic T, Breteau G, et al. Acute myelopathies: clinical, laboratory and outcome profiles in 79 cases. Brain 2001;124:1509–21.

86. Proposed diagnostic criteria and nosology of acute transverse myelitis. Neurology 2002;59:499–505.

87. Kesselring J, Miller DH, Robb SA, et al. Acute disseminated encephalomyelitis: MRI findings and the distinction from multiple sclerosis. Brain 1990;113: 291–302.

88. Miller DH, Scaravilli F, Thomas DC, et al. Acute disseminated encephalomyelitis presenting as a solitary brainstem mass. J Neurol Neurosurg Psychiatr 1993;56:920–2.

89. Sebastián de la Cruz F, La Banda BF, Romero GJ. [Acute nontraumatic myelopathies: a review of 36 cases]. Rev Clin Esp 1995;195:380–6 [Spanish].

90. Aldeeb SM, Yaqub BA, Bruyn GW, et al. Acute transverse myelitis: a localized form of postinfectious encephalomyelitis. Brain 1997;120:1115–22.

91. Mok CC, Lau CS, Chan ET, et al. Acute transverse myelopathy in systemic lupus erythematosus: clinical presentation, treatment, and outcome. J Rheumatol 1998;25:467–73.

92. Campi A, Filippi M, Comi G, et al. Acute transverse myelopathy: spinal and cranial MR study with clinical follow-up. Ajnr: American Journal of Neuroradiology 1995;16:115–23.

93. April RS, Vansonnenberg E. A case of neuromyelitis optica (Devic's syndrome) in systemic lupus erythematosus: clinicopathologic report and review of the literature. Neurology 1976;26:1066–70.

94. Gil-Neciga E, Salinas E, Arenas C. [Devic's optic neuromyelitis. Follow-up of the evolution of the medullary lesions using magnetic resonance]. Rev Neurol 1997;25:241–4 [Spanish].

95. Tartaglino LM, Croul SE, Flanders AE, et al. Idiopathic acute transverse myelitis: MR imaging findings. Radiology 1996;201:661–9.

96. Pradhan S, Gupta RK, Ghosh D. Parainfectious myelitis: three distinct clinico-imagiological patterns with prognostic implications. Acta Neurol Scand 1997;95:241–7.

97. Barkhof F, Scheltens P, Valk J, et al. Serial quantitative MR assessment of optic neuritis in a case of neuromyelitis optica, using Gadolinium-enhanced STIR imaging. Neuroradiology 1991;33:70–1.

98. Kovacs B, Lafferty TL, Brent LH, et al. Transverse myelopathy in systemic lupus erythematosus: an analysis of 14 cases and review of the literature. Ann Rheum Dis 2000;59:120–4.

99. Takahashi T, Fujihara K, Nakashima I, et al. Anti-aquaporin-4 antibody is involved in the pathogenesis of NMO: a study on antibody titre. Brain 2007;130:1235–43.

100. Lalive PH, Menge T, Barman I, et al. Identification of new serum autoantibodies in neuromyelitis optica using protein microarrays. Neurology 2006;67:176–7.

101. Misu T, Fujihara K, Kakita A, et al. Loss of aquaporin 4 in lesions of neuromyelitis optica: distinction from multiple sclerosis. Brain 2007;130:1224–34.

102. Roemer SF, Parisi JE, Lennon VA, et al. Pattern-specific loss of aquaporin-4 immunoreactivity distinguishes neuromyelitis optica from multiple sclerosis. Brain 2007;130:1194–205.

103. Wingerchuk DM, Lennon VA, Pittock SJ, et al. Revised diagnostic criteria for neuromyelitis optica. Neurology 2006;66:1485–9.

104. Dale RC, de SC, Chong WK, et al. Acute disseminated encephalomyelitis, multiphasic disseminated encephalomyelitis and multiple sclerosis in children. Brain 2000;123(Pt 12):2407–22.

105. Rovaris M, Inglese M, Viti B, et al. The contribution of fast-FLAIR MRI for lesion detection in the brain of patients with systemic autoimmune diseases. J Neurol 2000;247:29–33.

106. Polman CH, Reingold SC, Edan G, et al. Diagnostic criteria for multiple sclerosis: 2005 revisions to the "McDonald Criteria". Ann Neurol 2005;58:840–6.

107. Traboulsee AL, Li DK. The role of MRI in the diagnosis of multiple sclerosis. Adv Neurol 2006;98:125–46.

108. Tintore M, Rovira A, Martinez MJ, et al. Isolated demyelinating syndromes: comparison of different MR imaging criteria to predict conversion to clinically definite multiple sclerosis. AJNR Am J Neuroradiol 2000;21:702–6.

109. Charil A, Yousry TA, Rovaris M, et al. MRI and the diagnosis of multiple sclerosis: expanding the concept of "no better explanation". Lancet Neurol 2006;5:841–52.

110. Barkhof F, van Waesberghe JH, Filippi M, et al. T(1) hypointense lesions in secondary progressive multiple sclerosis: effect of interferon beta-1b treatment. Brain 2001;124:1396–402.

111. Mainero C, De SN, Iannucci G, et al. Correlates of MS disability assessed in vivo using aggregates of MR quantities. Neurology 2001;56:1331–4.

112. Filippi M. In-vivo tissue characterization of multiple sclerosis and other white matter diseases using magnetic resonance based techniques. J Neurol 2001;248:1019–29.

113. Filippi M, Bozzali M, Horsfield MA, et al. A conventional and magnetization transfer MRI study of the cervical cord in patients with MS. Neurology 2000;54:207–13.

114. Agosta F, Benedetti B, Rocca MA, et al. Quantification of cervical cord pathology in primary progressive MS using diffusion tensor MRI. Neurology 2005;64:631–5.

115. Valsasina P, Rocca MA, Agosta F, et al. Mean diffusivity and fractional anisotropy histogram analysis of the cervical cord in MS patients. Neuroimage 2005;26:822–8.

116. Valsasina P, Agosta F, Benedetti B, et al. Diffusion anisotropy of the cervical cord is strictly associated with disability in amyotrophic lateral sclerosis. J Neurol Neurosurg Psychiatr 2007;78:480–4.

117. Benedetti B, Valsasina P, Judica E, et al. Grading cervical cord damage in neuromyelitis optica and MS by diffusion tensor MRI. Neurology 2006;67:161–3.

118. Agosta F, Absinta M, Sormani MP, et al. In vivo assessment of cervical cord damage in MS patients: a longitudinal diffusion tensor MRI study. Brain 2007;130:2211–9.

119. Bjartmar C, Kidd G, Mork S, et al. Neurological disability correlates with spinal cord axonal loss and reduced N-acetyl aspartate in chronic multiple sclerosis patients. Ann Neurol 2000;48:893–901.

120. Kendi AT, Tan FU, Kendi M, et al. MR spectroscopy of cervical spinal cord in patients with multiple sclerosis. Neuroradiology 2004;46:764–9.

121. Marliani AF, Clementi V, bini-Riccioli L, et al. Quantitative proton magnetic resonance spectroscopy of the human cervical spinal cord at 3 Tesla. Magn Reson Med 2007;57:160–3.

122. Blamire AM, Cader S, Lee M, et al. Axonal damage in the spinal cord of multiple sclerosis patients detected by magnetic resonance spectroscopy. Magn Reson Med 2007;58:880–5.

123. Cooke FJ, Blamire AM, Manners DN, et al. Quantitative proton magnetic resonance spectroscopy of the cervical spinal cord. Magn Reson Med 2004; 51:1122–8.

124. Ciccarelli O, Wheeler-Kingshott CA, McLean MA, et al. Spinal cord spectroscopy and diffusion-based tractography to assess acute disability in multiple sclerosis. Brain 2007;130:2220–31.

125. Stroman PW, Krause V, Malisza KL, et al. Characterization of contrast changes in functional MRI of the human spinal cord at 1.5 T. Magn Reson Imaging 2001;19:833–8.

126. Stroman PW, Ryner LN. Functional MRI of motor and sensory activation in the human spinal cord. Magn Reson Imaging 2001;19:27–32.

127. Stroman PW, Tomanek B, Krause V, et al. Mapping of neuronal function in the healthy and injured human spinal cord with spinal fMRI. Neuroimage 2002;17:1854–60.

128. Stroman PW, Krause V, Malisza KL, et al. Extravascular proton-density changes as a non-BOLD component of contrast in fMRI of the human spinal cord. Magn Reson Med 2002;48: 122–7.

129. Stroman PW, Krause V, Malisza KL, et al. Functional magnetic resonance imaging of the human cervical spinal cord with stimulation of different sensory dermatomes. Magn Reson Imaging 2002;20:1–6.

130. Stroman PW. Magnetic resonance imaging of neuronal function in the spinal cord: spinal FMRI. Clin Med Res 2005;3:146–56.

131. Stroman PW, Kornelsen J, Lawrence J. An improved method for spinal functional MRI with large volume coverage of the spinal cord. J Magn Reson Imaging 2005;21:520–6.

132. Stroman PW. Discrimination of errors from neuronal activity in functional MRI of the human spinal cord by means of general linear model analysis. Magn Reson Med 2006;56:452–6.

133. Agosta F, Valsasina P, Caputo D, et al. Tactile-associated recruitment of the cervical cord is altered in patients with multiple sclerosis. Neuroimage 2008;39:1542–8.

134. Agosta F, Valsasina P, Rocca MA, et al. Evidence for enhanced functional activity of cervical cord in relapsing multiple sclerosis. Magn Reson Med 2008;59:1035–42.

Brain Imaging of Multiple Sclerosis: the Next 10 Years

Paul M. Matthews, DPhil, FRCP[a,b,*,1]

KEYWORDS

- MR imaging • Functional MR imaging
- Positron emission tomography • Multiple sclerosis
- Imaging • Myelin • Inflammation

Over the past 3 decades,[1] MR imaging has become a primary tool for the investigation of multiple sclerosis (MS) and for clinical diagnosis. A key milestone was passed with introduction of the McDonald criteria,[2] which established specific criteria for MR imaging–supported diagnosis. More recent criteria have expanded the applications, scope, and potential sensitivity to allow a reliable diagnosis to be made within a year of initial presentation, even without use of contrast agents.[3–5] This incorporation of MR imaging into routine clinical practice has been a major driver for past development of MS imaging.

Another driver has been the role of MR imaging as a disease activity and progression biomarker in new drug development.[6] MR imaging changes correlate well with neuropathologic features.[7,8] Many studies have confirmed correlations between acute gadolinium (Gd) enhancement of T1-weighted MR imaging and relapse or chronic structural changes (eg, brain atrophy) and clinical progression.[9–11] This has led to acceptance of MR imaging as a near surrogate marker in recent clinical trials of anti-inflammatory therapies for MS.

The development of new types of MR imaging contrast, advances in radiofrequency coil design, and the availability of higher magnet field strengths provide a greater range of imaging measures with higher sensitivity for neuropathologic changes and greater anatomic resolution.[12–14] The development of a wide range of software tools now widely disseminated publicly (eg,[15,16]) and commercially enables imagers with even limited specialist analytic resources to apply increasingly sophisticated approaches for quantitative data interpretation. Coupled to advances in information technology (IT), a new quantitative neuroradiology of MS has emerged. This already has had an impact on clinical trials.[10,17] It holds additional promise as an approach to improved precision of individual prognosis or assessments of clinical therapeutic responses.

Ten years is a surprisingly short time. This author is also aware of the difficulties of accurately looking to the future even this near, however. Nonetheless, current trends in imaging science suggest some specific types of applications development that appear likely. Potential advances in the application of MR imaging techniques are considered. The great opportunities for molecular imaging, particularly for increasing understanding of the dynamics of MS pathologic findings and in support of early development of neurotherapeutics, are outlined.

ADVANCES IN MR IMAGING
Toward the Goal of "Personalized Medicine"

One of the most striking features of MS is the heterogeneity of expression.[18] Heterogeneity of neuropathologic findings mirrors the heterogeneity in the clinical course. Lucchinetti and colleagues[19] have proposed four distinct pathologic forms of the disease. These differences suggest rational

a Glaxo Smith Kline Clinical Imaging Centre, Hammersmith Hospital, London, UK
b Department of Clinical Neurosciences, Imperial College, London, UK
1 The author is a full-time employee of GlaxoSmithKline.
* GlaxoSmithKline Clinical Imaging Centre, Hammersmith Hospital, London, UK.
E-mail address: paul.m.matthews@gsk.com

Neuroimag Clin N Am 19 (2009) 101–112
doi:10.1016/j.nic.2008.08.003
1052-5149/08/$ – see front matter © 2008 Elsevier Inc. All rights reserved.

hypotheses concerning the major differences in prognosis and responses to therapy that are likely to be tested in coming years. With increasing use of advanced imaging tools that allow coregistration of images acquired with different contrasts, explicitly multivariate analyses of regional pathologic changes are possible.[6,20–22] Classifiers based on these multivariate features can be used in vivo in ways that are similar to the ways in which conventional histologic stains are used ex vivo.

Stratification of patients on the basis of imaging neuropathologic findings (in combination with other approaches) should be explored for better targeting of treatments.[23] Differentiation of drugs in the market is a key goal for pharmaceutical companies.[24] Clear demonstrations of new drug value are being demanded by payers. In this environment, there is an opportunity to couple the use of imaging methods that speed proof of pharmacology in early drug development to stratification of responder populations. MS is an ideal "test case" for this new way of working, given the range of aspects of the disease process that can be imaged even now.[12]

A related aspect of personalized medicine is to define when treatments have achieved their goals or are no longer having a major impact on disease processes in individual patients. The clinical significance of neutralizing antibodies with interferon treatments, for example, can be resolved with more data relating the nature and magnitude of antibody responses and MR imaging–assessed new disease activity using standardized approaches.[25] Although serial MR imaging studies have not been an effective way of monitoring treatment in the past because of the relatively modest effects of the drugs, as more effective treatments become available,[26,27] quantitative criteria for determining treatment evaluation periods even for individual patients should be able to be formulated.

Harnessing the Power of Large Studies

A major enabler for an evidence-based quantitative approach to clinical decision making based on imaging neuropathologic findings is likely to be more large well-powered outcome studies. Because resources for new investigations are always limited, however, the opportunity to build these on a stronger foundation of imaging IT integration within health centers needs to be seized. Needs of imaging for clinical care and imaging for research evaluation of patients can be met together.[28] There is an increasing potential for standardization among even sophisticated imaging protocols.[29] Observational studies can be constructed based on data derived from other research activities or usual clinical practice. Although limited to submitted clinical trials data sets and centralized (rather than having archiving distributed at different centers providing data), the Sylvia Laurie Center provides a model of how this kind of activity can generate substantial new value,[30] although the statistical models used for studies must appropriately take into account the biases that can be introduced by this kind of retrospective databasing.[31]

The potential for this kind of "e-science" should be enhanced as electronic patient records are used more widely. The technical problems associated with large-scale electronic archiving of image data were solved over the past decade, and there already is widespread use of conventional picture archiving and communication (PACS) systems in filmless neuroradiology units. Improvements to the software environment and hardware capacities may be expected to enable full integration of these data with other patient records information in common databasing frameworks. This should allow clinical outcomes and imaging data to be related rapidly within any single institution.[28] With care to ensure that all personally identifiable information is removed, these data can be shared among researchers in different institutions to facilitate the kinds of large meta-analyses needed to understand trends in a heterogeneous disease.

More ambitious population-based imaging studies should become more common as this value for other types of disease epidemiology is realized. A recent study of extended families in Sardinia illustrates the value of this type of study, with the demonstration of significant expression of white matter abnormalities in asymptomatic first-degree relatives of patients who had MS.[32] Biobank efforts underway in several countries to chart the risk factors and extended prodromes for common diseases by long-term monitoring of extremely large (500,000+ persons) healthy populations should provide an entirely new kind of information.[33] Although thus far, these efforts have been directed toward follow-up of a middle-aged population, they may be expected to be expanded into earlier stages of the life cycle and into periods when the risks for developing MS are higher.

Software for high-quality unsupervised image analysis must be a major development focus to enable this type of work. Already, academic laboratories have developed tools that are relatively robust to minor variations in acquisition techniques,[34–36] allowing increasingly automated approaches to the derivation of specific metrics from imaging data sets. With some improvements, these should allow large archived primary data sources to be mined rapidly for specific metrics. Collaborative multicenter archiving should facilitate the discovery and qualification of measures with sufficient power to encourage their rapid acceptance by the imaging community.

Imaging Genomics

By increasing potential study size, all these developments allow a qualitatively new type of experiment. Plausibly sufficient power has become available for testing genetic hypotheses utilizing brain structural (and, potentially, functional) changes using imaging as an intermediate or "endo"-phenotype,[37] for which a greater proportion of population variance can be explained by single gene differences than with usual clinical features.

One recent study has provided evidence for an association between the brain-derived neurotrophic factor met66 allele and lower degrees of neocortical gray matter atrophy and T2 lesion volume in patients.[38] Another study has suggested a relation between functional polymorphisms in the CCR5 and CCO5 ligand/receptor pair and worse clinical disease course and altered T2 and T1 lesion loads on MR imaging.[39] The CCR5 303*G polymorphism was associated with reduced T2 hyperintense and T1 hypointense lesion volumes.

Critical review of these findings suggests that although of great interest, they need to be replicated before they can be accepted as more than hypotheses.[40] The numbers of plausible gene associations are huge across different disease subphenotypes. This brings considerable potential for false-positive results. What has been lacking thus far in the literature is a full understanding of the number of potential associations that have been tested before the finding of the individually significant changes reported. Much larger populations also are needed for confidence in outcomes, because the contributions of single genes can be expected to be heterogeneous.

Nonetheless, the approach is promising and is potentially a way of directly linking functional and structural imaging to molecular pathologic findings.[41] Obvious extensions of the single polymorphism genetic approach should involve the use of pathway analyses that assess whether clusters of genes with related functions are associated with a feature. Image analysis based on transcriptomic profiling also is to be expected.[42]

New Applications and New MR Imaging Contrast Agents

Preclinical studies have demonstrated the complex dynamics of inflammatory response and the potential for selective imaging of different cell populations and effector molecules. Expression of endothelial inflammatory mediators,[43] cell trafficking,[44] and macrophage infiltration[45,46] all can be imaged with targeted MR imaging contrast agents. With the development of immune therapies directed against specific aspects of the inflammatory cascade, these measures should ideally be extended to human studies to characterize the response across different clinical syndromes and to provide better pharmacodynamic measures for early-phase drug development.

Ultrasmall iron oxide (FeO) particles have been approved for other indications. Their dextran coating is associated with only a modest rate of (largely minor) adverse events, and more biologically inert alternatives can be expected.[47] Injected particles are engulfed by circulating monocytes before they migrate into a new inflammatory lesion (compelling direct evidence, which has been presented with studies of carotid plaques).[46] The contrast thus provides an index of the dynamics of a specific arm of the antigen-presenting inflammatory cell pool. It provides information complementary to Gd MR imaging, which reports on changes in blood-brain barrier permeability probably reflecting an earlier stage of evolution of a focal lesion.[48]

In principle, lymphocytes could be labeled ex vivo and reinjected, but this kind of experiment is complex and raises safety issues that may be difficult to resolve in a research context. Unfortunately, despite the availability of antibodies directed against surface proteins specific for particular immune cell populations (eg, rituximab) and surface determinants, the potential for widespread use of similar molecules with Gd or FeO labels seems modest. The relatively low sensitivity of conventional MR imaging contrast is one major issue, particularly given that any contrast would need to be administered in low enough doses to preclude significant biologic activity. Amplification of contrast signal[49] or use of ultra-high-field imaging[50] could present a solution, however. A specific concern with antibody-based targeting is that the contrast agent has sufficiently rapid kinetics to clear the blood pool fast enough to allow selective tissue imaging, although this could be managed by appropriate re-engineering.[51] The hurdle of ensuring safety for subjects with such pharmacologically complex agents remains.

Extending the Understanding of Axonal Pathologic Findings

Diffusion MR imaging
A rediscovery of the importance of axonal injury in MS in the 1990s[52] and new recognition of its

potentially critical importance in determining disability[53-55] should undoubtedly lead to further developments in quantitative axonal structural imaging over the next decade.

Diffusion tensor MR imaging is now a well-accepted tool for mapping structural connectivity among brain regions.[56] The fractional anisotropy that characterizes white matter has components that can be related to restricted diffusion of water associated with myelin and with the axoplasm.[57,58] Diffusion measures are sensitive to demyelination, axonal loss, and probably also to the changes in caliber and axonal internal organization[59] associated with demyelination. Developments in instrumentation and analytic tools[60] are making it much easier to obtain exceptionally high-quality diffusion MR imaging data that can be related directly to anatomic features of white matter[61-63] and gray matter.[64-66]

A major issue that has limited development in the field has been accurately comparing myelin organization between individuals and groups. Conventional software tools for brain registration perform white matter registration poorly because of the lack of specific contrast edges to drive anatomically meaningful landmark matching. One advance has been to use tract-based spatial statistics (TBSS).[67] This simple approach uses the fractional anisotropy within an individual brain to develop a white matter "skeleton" reflecting major local trends that can be used as a registration framework. Quantitative variations in the skeleton can be used to contrast spatial changes in white matter across individuals and groups, defining variation in robust statistical terms, and thereby establishing potential diagnostic and prognostic criteria.

An alternative approach has been to characterize changes within anatomically defined white matter.[68,69] Although this approach is more user-intensive, automation should be possible. Exploration of the distribution of connectivity measures within individual tracts can define potentially sensitive and specific neuropathologic measures.[68,70] The advantages of diffusion MR imaging lie in the sensitivity to microstructural changes.[58]

Proton magnetic resonance spectroscopy

Axonal pathologic findings also can be defined metabolically.[6,71] Proton magnetic resonance spectroscopy was the first approach in the modern era to highlight the considerable extent of neuroaxonal injury in the disease. The N-acetyl aspartate (NAA) resonance reflects mitochondrial function.[72,73] Mitochondria may be impaired early in inflammatory response by immune modulators, such as nitric oxide.[74] There have been suggestions in the literature over the past decade that metabolic changes in the disease are early,[75-77] precede irreversible loss of axons,[78] and may be reversible.[77] These concepts should be tested and developed further over the next decade.

One report has shown recovery of reduced NAA after introduction of interferon-β treatment.[79] This suggests that neuronal metabolism is improved by reducing inflammation. Reversible neuroaxonal mitochondrial metabolic dysfunction also has been reported in other diseases.[80] Much more needs to be done to develop this exciting notion, however.[78] A first small follow-up study was unable to reproduce the finding with interferon-β, suggesting that there is variation in patient response-related factors, such as disease stage or subtype.[81]

Greater Focus on the Gray Matter

It now is well accepted that gray matter is involved extensively in MS. Demyelinating lesions are common in the cortex and subcortical gray matter.[82,83] Extended fields of subpial demyelination also can be found across the cortex. These are likely related to nodules of B-cell infiltration in the overlying meninges[84,85] and may reflect action of diffusing anti-myelin antibodies. Atrophy of cortical[83,86] and subcortical[76,87] gray matter has been well demonstrated and is progressive through the disease. In the neocortex, this may largely be attributable to a relative neurite dystrophy,[83,88,89] but in the subcortical nuclei, such as the thalamus, atrophy is associated with substantial loss of neurons.[87]

Conventional imaging approaches only rarely visualize gray matter inflammatory lesions. This seems, in part, to be a consequence of altered relative reduced contrast between the inflammatory lesions and normal gray matter.[90] Inversion recovery sequences contribute to usable contrast with efforts to improve signal-to-noise with greater image averaging. Limited resolution of conventional images for the thin (2.5 mm or so) neocortex also plays a role, however, and may be expected to be addressed further in the future with use of high-field systems and high-resolution scanning protocols.[91] New imaging sequences are being developed in several laboratories (eg, high-resolution T1 mapping techniques).[92] Further developments are expected.

Because the problem of resolution critically depends on signal-to-noise, the recent availability of 7.0-T imaging for humans may open up new potential for cortical imaging of MS lesions. Recent data suggest that linear in-plane resolution on the order of 250 μm or better should be achievable commonly at this field.[12,50] Advantages may accrue from the ability to visualize the close relation between small draining veins and inflammatory lesions.

Improved analytic tools should continue to have significant impact for studies of gray matter. Better methods for segmentation of gray matter particularly should help to drive the field forward. If the need for time-consuming manual interventions can be reduced, cortical flattening methods should greatly enable more sensitive quantitative assessment of gray matter changes.[93,94] The correlations between disability progression and brain atrophy[95] and between brain atrophy and gray matter loss[86] suggest that clinically relevant prognostic measures could be derived. Extensions of the paradigm for cognition also seem possible.[96]

New Range of Clinical-Pathophysiologic Correlations

Perfusion MR imaging

Integrating neuropathologic information into clinically meaningful outcome measures should be enhanced by the use of different types of physiologic summary measures. These can assess tissue function as it is affected by the neuropathologic findings. Brain perfusion provides one such measure. The past few years have seen substantial developments in this area, with availability of robust sequences for noninvasive arterial spin tagging and methods for quantitation of the perfusion changes.[97] Pilot studies have demonstrated that cerebral blood flow is reduced in brains of patients who have MS, consistent with prior positron emission tomography (PET) studies.[98] Perfusion is increased in acute inflammatory foci, however. The arterial spin labeling techniques should be enhanced by the availability of improved flow-sensitive sequences, higher signal-to-noise with phased-array coils, and higher field MR imaging.[99,100] One goal is to use perfusion MR imaging as a marker "intermediate" between measures of neuropathologic and clinical outcomes. As a measure of function, perfusion MR imaging provides indices of the consequences of pathologic findings, not just locally but in functionally connected regions of brain.[101]

Functional MR imaging

The past several years have also seen growth in applications of functional MR (fMR) imaging to MS.[102–107] fMR imaging is an indirect measure of aggregate excitation-inhibition in gray matter microcircuits.[108] Perhaps the most important outcome of fMR imaging studies in MS over the past several years has been to highlight brain circuit plasticity and its potentially adaptive role.[109,110] An argument for the importance of adaptive plasticity as a limit to expression of the neuropathologic findings is particularly compelling for this disease in which irreversible neuroaxonal changes accompany even the early acute inflammatory responses, whereas patients show complete clinical recoveries after relapses. Potentially maladaptive functional changes may be seen, however.[111,112] Progressive disease pathologic findings also must limit the potential for adaptive capacity.[113,114]

Although precise interpretation of fMR imaging measures is still needed, fMR imaging applications are likely to grow substantially. Spinal cord fMR imaging has been demonstrated convincingly[115] and promises the potential to assess relative contributions of plasticity at the spinal and cerebral levels to recovery. The approach offers a potential way of objectively assessing neurorehabilitation[116,117] or other therapies that promote plasticity.[118,119] Pilot applications suggest the possible utility of extensions of the univariate analytic approaches (regional functional activation measures) to multivariate (eg, functional connectivity) measures that may provide more powerful measures of longer distance integration of brain systems.[114,120,121] Encouragingly for applications to the evaluation of therapies, recent work has demonstrated how fMR imaging can be applied with confidence in multicenter protocols.[29,122]

Myelin repair

Magnetization transfer ratio and short T2 imaging The past 3 decades have focused attention in MR imaging studies on the primary inflammatory events and their immediate sequelae. A major goal now is to extend understanding of tissue repair and, particularly, remyelination.

Several studies have now provided compelling demonstrations that multicompartment T2 relaxation provides relatively specific information on myelin content from the short T2 component of the brain water MR imaging signal that is thought to reflect water associated closely with myelin.[123] The extent of local changes in myelin water content with demyelination is large (30%–50%) within macroscopic MR imaging voxels.[124] This suggests that measurement of the myelin water fraction should be viable as a measure of remyelination for assessment of therapies directed at enhancing intrinsic remyelination pathways or at stem cell replacement therapies. Thus far, however, the technique has not been widely used. A major limitation was that only single-slice acquisition was practical.[125] New applications should expand with the availability of multislice or three-dimensional acquisition techniques that allow whole-brain coverage.

Magnetization transfer (MT) MR imaging is an alternative method for assessing characteristics of the water pool associated with myelin.[126] It is sensitive to early changes that can precede the development of Gd-enhancing lesions by many months, and therefore must reflect microscopic pathologic findings of myelin.[21] MT MR imaging (which typically uses whole-brain acquisition) has been related to the evolution of lesions longitudinally in many studies. As expected from the sensitivity to demyelination, MT MR imaging seems sensitive to early remyelination. Chen and colleagues[127] have provided data recently suggesting that the dynamics of remyelination can be monitored quantitatively in individual lesions over the days to weeks after acute relapse. Future research needs to assess whether patterns of recovery in individual patients provide a good prognostic measure and whether the nature of the remyelination response is a useful index of underlying pathologic mechanisms[19] for patient stratification. MT MR imaging also should enable development of remyelination therapies by providing a powerful pharmacodynamic outcome measure for clinical trials.

The two approaches to myelin imaging rely on different contrast mechanisms, and therefore are complementary. Their relative sensitivity and specificity need further exploration. In addition, although substantial qualification has been possible using postmortem material, both rely on making inferences about relations between molecular dynamics reflected in biophysical phenomena and pathologic findings that are indirect. Availability of a specifically targeted molecular imaging marker of myelin would be ideal.[128]

Molecular imaging Another route to an improved understanding of the dynamic molecular pathologic findings of MS is to make use of exquisitely sensitive PET methods to characterize molecular changes directly. PET has been applied for some years for metabolic studies in MS and in other many neurologic diseases.[129] The cerebral metabolic rate for oxidation of the preferred brain substrate, glucose (CMR_{glu}), can be measured with injection of positron-emitting ^{18}F-2-fluro-2-deoxy-D-glucose (FDG). Brain oxidative metabolism is coupled closely to the closely coupled neuronal and glial metabolic changes associated with neurotransmitter release. In patients who have MS, reductions in the global metabolic rate for glucose are most pronounced in the prefrontal cortex and in specific subcortical regions, including the hippocampus and thalamus.[130] Progressive reductions are seen over time, suggesting a close relation between metabolism and the changes in

neuronal activity contributing to longer term disability.[131,132]

Focal inflammatory lesions show increased glucose metabolism as a consequence of the increased glycolytic rates of inflammatory cells.[133] These changes can be defined in white matter and are associated with acute relapses. Molecularly specific measures of the focal immune response also are possible because of the high sensitivity of PET. PK11195 is an isoquinoline that binds relatively specifically to the peripheral benzodiazepine receptor (PBR; translocator protein 18KDa).[134] PBR is an outer membrane protein of mitochondria that is located predominantly in glial cells (astrocytes and microglia). Increased PK11195 binding reflecting increased PBR protein expression is found in MS. This up-regulation may reflect an increase in mitochondrial number or an increase in the number of PBR sites of mitochondria with activation of cells. In practice, it may be able to be interpreted as a marker for activated microglia in the brain.

A pilot study demonstrated uptake of PK11195 within the sites of active MS lesions defined by MR imaging.[135] More comprehensive follow-up with in vitro pathologic correlations indicated that although increases in PBR expression were found in regions of focal inflammatory pathologic change, changes also were seen in the cerebral gray matter and projection areas of lesioned white matter, which is potentially consistent with a microglial reaction after axonal transection.[136]

Additional tracer molecules have been described that also bind to the PBR receptor (eg, PBR28, vinpocetine) but that have potentially more favorable imaging characteristics.[137,138] Robust interpretation of results demands validation of modeling methods for specific signal detection. These are now being better defined.[138] Over the next 10 years, the applications of these molecules for understanding the nature of the innate immune response in MS should thus increase. This should open up new potential for assessment of the effects of therapeutically targeting microglia.

This is only one of several types of molecular targets that should help us to understand the pathologic findings of this disease, however. PET has an increasing potential for defining pathologic findings in a specific neuronal population, which may allow differentiation of individual neuronal subclasses based on such features as neurotransmitter receptor distribution. Histopathologic evidence has suggested selective neuronal vulnerability in MS; smaller axons seem to be more susceptible to damage.[139] The hypothesis that GABAergic signaling[140] is relatively selectively reduced in cortical lesions of MS can be tested directly using receptor probes, such as flumazenil.[141,142] Information related to this could be used to suggest modulatory neurotransmitter treatments that might modify symptoms or, if PET measures were extended to stem cell–specific markers, the integration of stem cells after transplantation.

Direct myelin imaging is a goal that should be achievable in the short term. Congo red–based molecules bind to myelin with a relative specificity that suggests their possible use as myelin PET tracers.[128] An initial set of studies has shown practicality for in vivo assessment and good specificity and sensitivity to MS-associated demyelination in vitro. What is needed now is further characterization of binding sites to allow accurate interpretation of changes in binding potential. It should be possible to develop tracers directed against more than one myelin component to get better insight into myelin structure-function changes with MS. Absolute quantitation of the PET signal is possible. Although the PET experiment is always going to be more expensive and invasive than MR imaging, this offers a way of "calibrating" indirect MR imaging measures in smaller experimental medicine studies.

A new era of imaging may be heralded by imaging agents that are developed in parallel with innovative therapies and have the potential to answer critical questions related to the proof of pharmacology (eg, labeled stabilized antisense oligonucleotides that could be used to assess delivery and half-life of the cognate therapeutic molecules).[143] Potentially therapeutic antibody fragments (eg, domain antibodies) can be labeled with a variety of positron-emitting isotopes and have kinetic characteristics favorable to imaging.[51,144] Because of the exquisite selectivity with which they can be targeted and their high affinity, these and similar antibody-related molecules may provide ideal ways of labeling individual cell populations. Although substantial technical hurdles remain, this would provide a way of "tagging" cells to study their trafficking and their longer term distribution in the body. This would enable studies evaluating those immune-modulatory agents directed against the ways in which individual cell populations migrate.

SUMMARY

Technology enabling new advances in MS imaging should continue to evolve over the next decade. There have been advances in MR imaging systems with the increasing availability of very-high-field magnets and more sensitive phased-array systems that promise increased resolution to the extent that new anatomic territories, such as the cortex, should able to be studied with precision. Wider availability of PET and enabling chemistry promises expansion of opportunities for molecular imaging. A particularly exciting prospect is the use of tagged biologic molecules that may couple the sensitivity of PET with exquisite molecular selectivity.

There are multiple drivers for applications of these improving technologies to imaging of MS, including the following:

1. Improved understanding of disease mechanisms
2. More efficient development of new medicines
3. Improved prognostication for patients
4. More efficient allocation of costly treatments

The next 10 years is thus undoubtedly likely to see exciting continued expansion of the role of neuroimaging in applications related to MS. This disease remains a powerful model for establishing the value of brain imaging for research, clinical applications, and therapeutics development.

The new imaging techniques, particularly those involving ultra-high-field MR imaging or PET, are costly, however. Emphasis on large-scale studies with more conventional techniques demands more substantial resources and cooperation. The new brain imaging science of the next decade should therefore place a premium on new kinds of partnerships between academic research groups, health care providers, and industry to deliver on the promise of imaging methods.

ACKNOWLEDGMENTS

The author gratefully acknowledges support from the Medical Research Council and from the MS Society of Great Britain and Northern Ireland for work conducted at the University of Oxford.

REFERENCES

1. Young IR, Hall AS, Pallis CA, et al. Nuclear magnetic resonance imaging of the brain in multiple sclerosis. Lancet 1981;2(8255):1063–6.
2. McDonald WI, Compston A, Edan G, et al. Recommended diagnostic criteria for multiple sclerosis: guidelines from the International Panel on the Diagnosis of Multiple Sclerosis. Ann Neurol 2001;50(1):121–7.
3. Miller DH, Filippi M, Fazekas F, et al. Role of magnetic resonance imaging within diagnostic criteria for multiple sclerosis. Ann Neurol 2004;56(2):273–8.
4. Korteweg T, Barkhof F, Uitdehaag BM, et al. How to use spinal cord magnetic resonance imaging in the

McDonald diagnostic criteria for multiple sclerosis. Ann Neurol 2005;57(4):606–7.

5. Polman CH, Reingold SC, Edan G, et al. Diagnostic criteria for multiple sclerosis: 2005 revisions to the "McDonald Criteria." Ann Neurol 2005;58(6):840–6.

6. Caramanos Z, Matthews PM, Arnold DL. Axonal pathology in patients with multiple sclerosis: evidence from in vivo proton magnetic resonance spectroscopy. In: Cohen J, Rudick R, editors. Multiple sclerosis therapeutics. Boca Raton (FL): CRC Press.

7. Bo L, Geurts JJ, Ravid R, et al. Magnetic resonance imaging as a tool to examine the neuropathology of multiple sclerosis. Neuropathol Appl Neurobiol 2004;30(2):106–17.

8. Lycklama a Nijeholt G, Barkhof F. Differences between subgroups of MS: MRI findings and correlation with histopathology. J Neurol Sci 2003;206(2):173–4.

9. Smith ME, Stone LA, Albert PS, et al. Clinical worsening in multiple sclerosis is associated with increased frequency and area of gadopentetate dimeglumine-enhancing magnetic resonance imaging lesions. Ann Neurol 1993;33(5):480–9.

10. Arnold DL, Matthews PM. MRI in the diagnosis and management of multiple sclerosis. Neurology 2002; 58(8 Suppl 4):S23–31.

11. Fisniku LK, Chard DT, Jackson JS, et al. Gray matter atrophy is related to long-term disability in multiple sclerosis. Ann Neurol 2008;63(3):247–54.

12. Bakshi R, Thompson AJ, Rocca MA, et al. MRI in multiple sclerosis: current status and future prospects. Lancet Neurol 2008;7(7):615–25.

13. Hickman SJ. Optic nerve imaging in multiple sclerosis. J Neuroimaging 2007;17(Suppl 1):42S–5S.

14. Wattjes MP, Lutterbey GG, Harzheim M, et al. Higher sensitivity in the detection of inflammatory brain lesions in patients with clinically isolated syndromes suggestive of multiple sclerosis using high field MRI: an intraindividual comparison of 1.5 T with 3.0 T. Eur Radiol 2006;16(9):2067–73.

15. Available at: www.fmrib.ox.ac.uk/fsl/. Accessed October 17, 2008.

16. Available at: www.fil.ion.ucl.ac.uk/spm/. Accessed October 17, 2008.

17. Kieseier BC, Wiendl H, Hemmer B, et al. Treatment and treatment trials in multiple sclerosis. Curr Opin Neurol 2007;20(3):286–93.

18. Confavreux C, Vukusic S. Natural history of multiple sclerosis: a unifying concept. Brain 2006;129(Pt 3): 606–16.

19. Lucchinetti C, Bruck W, Parisi J, et al. Heterogeneity of multiple sclerosis lesions: implications for the pathogenesis of demyelination. Ann Neurol 2000; 47(6):707–17.

20. Pathak SD, Ng L, Wyman B, et al. Quantitative image analysis: software systems in drug development trials. Drug Discov Today 2003;8(10): 451–8.

21. Pike GB, De Stefano N, Narayanan S, et al. Multiple sclerosis: magnetization transfer MR imaging of white matter before lesion appearance on T2-weighted images. Radiology 2000;215(3):824–30.

22. Wu Y, Warfield SK, Tan IL, et al. Automated segmentation of multiple sclerosis lesion subtypes with multichannel MRI. Neuroimage 2006;32(3): 1205–15.

23. Trusheim MR, Berndt ER, Douglas FL. Stratified medicine: strategic and economic implications of combining drugs and clinical biomarkers. Nat Rev Drug Discov 2007;6(4):287–93.

24. Booth B, Zemmel R. Quest for the best. Nat Rev Drug Discov 2003;2(10):838–41.

25. Fox EJ, Vartanian TK, Zamvil SS. The immunogenicity of disease-modifying therapies for multiple sclerosis: clinical implications for neurologists. Neurologist 2007;13(6):355–62.

26. Coles AJ, Wing MG, Molyneux P, et al. Monoclonal antibody treatment exposes three mechanisms underlying the clinical course of multiple sclerosis. Ann Neurol 1999;46(3):296–304.

27. Polman CH, O'Connor PW, Havrdova E, et al. A randomized, placebo-controlled trial of natalizumab for relapsing multiple sclerosis. N Engl J Med 2006;354(9):899–910.

28. Liu L, Meier D, Polgar-Turcsanyi M, et al. Multiple sclerosis medical image analysis and information management. J Neuroimaging 2005;15(4 Suppl): 103S–17S.

29. Bosnell R, Wegner C, Kincses ZT, et al. Reproducibility of fMRI in the clinical setting: implications for trial designs. Neuroimage 2008.

30. Held U, Heigenhauser L, Shang C, et al. Predictors of relapse rate in MS clinical trials. Neurology 2005; 65(11):1769–73.

31. Schach S, Scholz M, Wolinsky JS, et al. Pooled historical MRI data as a basis for research in multiple sclerosis—a statistical evaluation. Mult Scler 2007; 13(4):509–16.

32. De Stefano N, Cocco E, Lai M, et al. Imaging brain damage in first-degree relatives of sporadic and familial multiple sclerosis. Ann Neurol 2006;59(4): 634–9.

33. Ollier W, Sprosen T, Peakman T. UK Biobank: from concept to reality. Pharmacogenomics 2005;6(6): 639–46.

34. Smith SM, Zhang Y, Jenkinson M, et al. Accurate, robust, and automated longitudinal and cross-sectional brain change analysis. Neuroimage 2002;17(1):479–89.

35. Stevenson VL, Smith SM, Matthews PM, et al. Monitoring disease activity and progression in primary progressive multiple sclerosis using MRI: sub-voxel registration to identify lesion changes and to detect cerebral atrophy. J Neurol 2002; 249(2):171–7.

36. Smith SM, Rao A, De Stefano N, et al. Longitudinal and cross-sectional analysis of atrophy in Alzheimer's disease: cross-validation of BSI, SIENA and SIENAX. Neuroimage 2007;36(4):1200–6.

37. Gottesman II, Gould TD. The endophenotype concept in psychiatry: etymology and strategic intentions. Am J Psychiatry 2003;160(4):636–45.

38. Zivadinov R, Weinstock-Guttman B, Benedict R, et al. Preservation of gray matter volume in multiple sclerosis patients with the Met allele of the rs6265 (Val66Met) SNP of brain-derived neurotrophic factor. Hum Mol Genet 2007;16(22):2659–68.

39. van Veen T, Nielsen J, Berkhof J, et al. CCL5 and CCR5 genotypes modify clinical, radiological and pathological features of multiple sclerosis. J Neuroimmunol 2007;190(1–2):157–64.

40. Chanock SJ, Manolio T, Boehnke M, et al. Replicating genotype-phenotype associations. Nature 2007;447(7145):655–60.

41. Meyer-Lindenberg A, Weinberger DR. Intermediate phenotypes and genetic mechanisms of psychiatric disorders. Nat Rev Neurosci 2006; 7(10):818–27.

42. Sturzebecher S, Wandinger KP, Rosenwald A, et al. Expression profiling identifies responder and non-responder phenotypes to interferon-beta in multiple sclerosis. Brain 2003;126(Pt 6):1419–29.

43. Sibson NR, Blamire AM, Bernades-Silva M, et al. MRI detection of early endothelial activation in brain inflammation. Magn Reson Med 2004;51(2): 248–52.

44. Bulte JW, Duncan ID, Frank JA. In vivo magnetic resonance tracking of magnetically labeled cells after transplantation. J Cereb Blood Flow Metab 2002;22(8):899–907.

45. Trivedi RA, Mallawarachi C, U-king-Im JM, et al. Identifying inflamed carotid plaques using in vivo USPIO-enhanced MR imaging to label plaque macrophages. Arterioscler Thromb Vasc Biol 2006;26(7):1601–6.

46. Trivedi RA, U-king-Im JM, Graves MJ, et al. In vivo detection of macrophages in human carotid atheroma: temporal dependence of ultrasmall superparamagnetic particles of iron oxide-enhanced MRI. Stroke 2004;35(7):1631–5.

47. Bellin MF, Roy C, Kinkel K, et al. Lymph node metastases: safety and effectiveness of MR imaging with ultrasmall superparamagnetic iron oxide particles—initial clinical experience. Radiology 1998; 207(3):799–808.

48. Dousset V, Brochet B, Deloire MS, et al. MR imaging of relapsing multiple sclerosis patients using ultra-small-particle iron oxide and compared with gadolinium. AJNR Am J Neuroradiol 2006;27(5): 1000–5.

49. Querol M, Bogdanov A Jr. Amplification strategies in MR imaging: activation and accumulation of sensing contrast agents (SCAs). J Magn Reson Imaging 2006;24(5):971–82.

50. Ge Y, Zohrabian VM, Grossman RI. Seven-tesla magnetic resonance imaging: new vision of microvascular abnormalities in multiple sclerosis. Arch Neurol 2008;65(6):812–6.

51. Olafsen T, Kenanova VE, Wu AM. Tunable pharmacokinetics: modifying the in vivo half-life of antibodies by directed mutagenesis of the Fc fragment. Nat Protoc 2006;1(4):2048–60.

52. Arnold DL, Matthews PM, Francis G, et al. Proton magnetic resonance spectroscopy of human brain in vivo in the evaluation of multiple sclerosis: assessment of the load of disease. Magn Reson Med 1990;14(1):154–9.

53. Fu L, Matthews PM, De Stefano N, et al. Imaging axonal damage of normal-appearing white matter in multiple sclerosis. Brain 1998;121(Pt 1):103–13.

54. De Stefano N, Matthews PM, Fu L, et al. Axonal damage correlates with disability in patients with relapsing-remitting multiple sclerosis. Results of a longitudinal magnetic resonance spectroscopy study. Brain 1998;121(Pt 8):1469–77.

55. Matthews PM, De Stefano N, Narayanan S, et al. Putting magnetic resonance spectroscopy studies in context: axonal damage and disability in multiple sclerosis. Semin Neurol 1998;18(3):327–36.

56. Ramnani N, Behrens TE, Penny W, et al. New approaches for exploring anatomical and functional connectivity in the human brain. Biol Psychiatry 2004;56(9):613–9.

57. Song SK, Yoshino J, Le TQ, et al. Demyelination increases radial diffusivity in corpus callosum of mouse brain. Neuroimage 2005;26(1):132–40.

58. Song SK, Sun SW, Ju WK, et al. Diffusion tensor imaging detects and differentiates axon and myelin degeneration in mouse optic nerve after retinal ischemia. Neuroimage 2003;20(3):1714–22.

59. Zhu B, Moore GR, Zwimpfer TJ, et al. Axonal cytoskeleton changes in experimental optic neuritis. Brain Res 1999;824(2):204–17.

60. Behrens TE, Woolrich MW, Jenkinson M, et al. Characterization and propagation of uncertainty in diffusion-weighted MR imaging. Magn Reson Med 2003;50(5):1077–88.

61. Wakana S, Jiang H, Nagae-Poetscher LM, et al. Fiber tract-based atlas of human white matter anatomy. Radiology 2004;230(1):77–87.

62. Catani M, Jones DK, ffytche DH. Perisylvian language networks of the human brain. Ann Neurol 2005;57(1):8–16.

63. Schmahmann JD, Pandya DN. Cerebral white matter—historical evolution of facts and notions concerning the organization of the fiber pathways of the brain. J Hist Neurosci 2007;16(3):237–67.

64. Tomassini V, Jbabdi S, Klein JC, et al. Diffusion-weighted imaging tractography-based parcellation

of the human lateral premotor cortex identifies dorsal and ventral subregions with anatomical and functional specializations. J Neurosci 2007;27(38): 10259–69.

65. Johansen-Berg H, Behrens TE, Robson MD, et al. Changes in connectivity profiles define functionally distinct regions in human medial frontal cortex. Proc Natl Acad Sci U S A 2004;101(36):13335–40.

66. Behrens TE, Johansen-Berg H, Woolrich MW, et al. Non-invasive mapping of connections between human thalamus and cortex using diffusion imaging. Nat Neurosci 2003;6(7):750–7.

67. Smith SM, Jenkinson M, Johansen-Berg H, et al. Tract-based spatial statistics: voxelwise analysis of multi-subject diffusion data. Neuroimage 2006; 31(4):1487–505.

68. Ciccarelli O, Behrens TE, Altmann DR, et al. Probabilistic diffusion tractography: a potential tool to assess the rate of disease progression in amyotrophic lateral sclerosis. Brain 2006;129(Pt 7):1859–71.

69. Ciccarelli O, Toosy AT, Hickman SJ, et al. Optic radiation changes after optic neuritis detected by tractography-based group mapping. Hum Brain Mapp 2005;25(3):308–16.

70. Ciccarelli O, Behrens TE, Johansen-Berg H, et al. Investigation of white matter pathology in ALS and PLS using tract-based spatial statistics. Hum Brain Mapp 2008, in press.

71. Matthews PM, Andermann F, Arnold DL. A proton magnetic resonance spectroscopy study of focal epilepsy in humans. Neurology 1990;40(6):985–9.

72. Moffett JR, Ross B, Arun P, et al. N-acetylaspartate in the CNS: from neurodiagnostics to neurobiology. Prog Neurobiol 2007;81(2):89–131.

73. Dautry C, Vaufrey F, Brouillet E, et al. Early N-acetylaspartate depletion is a marker of neuronal dysfunction in rats and primates chronically treated with the mitochondrial toxin 3-nitropropionic acid. J Cereb Blood Flow Metab 2000;20(5):789–99.

74. Smith KJ, Lassmann H. The role of nitric oxide in multiple sclerosis. Lancet Neurol 2002;1(4):232–41.

75. De Stefano N, Narayanan S, Francis GS, et al. Evidence of axonal damage in the early stages of multiple sclerosis and its relevance to disability. Arch Neurol 2001;58(1):65–70.

76. Wylezinska M, Cifelli A, Jezzard P, et al. Thalamic neurodegeneration in relapsing-remitting multiple sclerosis. Neurology 2003;60(12):1949–54.

77. De Stefano N, Matthews PM, Arnold DL. Reversible decreases in N-acetylaspartate after acute brain injury. Magn Reson Med 1995;34(5):721–7.

78. Cader S, Johansen-Berg H, Wylezinska M, et al. Discordant white matter N-acetylaspartate and diffusion MRI measures suggest that chronic metabolic dysfunction contributes to axonal pathology in multiple sclerosis. Neuroimage 2007;36(1):19–27.

79. Narayanan S, De Stefano N, Francis GS, et al. Axonal metabolic recovery in multiple sclerosis patients treated with interferon beta-1b. J Neurol 2001;248(11):979–86.

80. Kalra S, Cashman NR, Genge A, et al. Recovery of N-acetylaspartate in corticomotor neurons of patients with ALS after riluzole therapy. Neuroreport 1998;9(8):1757–61.

81. Parry A, Corkill R, Blamire AM, et al. Beta-interferon treatment does not always slow the progression of axonal injury in multiple sclerosis. J Neurol 2003; 250(2):171–8.

82. Peterson JW, Bo L, Mork S, et al. Transected neurites, apoptotic neurons, and reduced inflammation in cortical multiple sclerosis lesions. Ann Neurol 2001;50(3):389–400.

83. Wegner C, Esiri MM, Chance SA, et al. Neocortical neuronal, synaptic, and glial loss in multiple sclerosis. Neurology 2006;67(6):960–7.

84. Pomeroy IM, Matthews PM, Frank JA, et al. Demyelinated neocortical lesions in marmoset autoimmune encephalomyelitis mimic those in multiple sclerosis. Brain 2005;128(Pt 11):2713–21.

85. Magliozzi R, Howell O, Vora A, et al. Meningeal B-cell follicles in secondary progressive multiple sclerosis associate with early onset of disease and severe cortical pathology. Brain 2007;130(Pt 4): 1089–104.

86. Chen JT, Narayanan S, Collins DL, et al. Relating neocortical pathology to disability progression in multiple sclerosis using MRI. Neuroimage 2004; 23(3):1168–75.

87. Cifelli A, Arridge M, Jezzard P, et al. Thalamic neurodegeneration in multiple sclerosis. Ann Neurol 2002;52(5):650–3.

88. Zhu B, Luo L, Moore GR, et al. Dendritic and synaptic pathology in experimental autoimmune encephalomyelitis. Am J Pathol 2003;162(5):1639–50.

89. Wegner C, Matthews PM. A new view of the cortex, new insights into multiple sclerosis. Brain 2003; 126(Pt 8):1719–21.

90. Bagnato F, Butman JA, Gupta S, et al. In vivo detection of cortical plaques by MR imaging in patients with multiple sclerosis. AJNR Am J Neuroradiol 2006;27(10):2161–7.

91. Bridge H, Clare S, Jenkinson M, et al. Independent anatomical and functional measures of the V1/V2 boundary in human visual cortex. J Vis 2005;5(2): 93–102.

92. Deoni SC, Peters TM, Rutt BK. High-resolution T1 and T2 mapping of the brain in a clinically acceptable time with DESPOT1 and DESPOT2. Magn Reson Med 2005;53(1):237–41.

93. Fischl B, Sereno MI, Dale AM. Cortical surface-based analysis. II: inflation, flattening, and a surface-based coordinate system. Neuroimage 1999; 9(2):195–207.

94. Dale AM, Fischl B, Sereno MI. Cortical surface-based analysis. I. Segmentation and surface reconstruction. Neuroimage 1999;9(2):179–94.

95. De Stefano N, Matthews PM, Filippi M, et al. Evidence of early cortical atrophy in MS: relevance to white matter changes and disability. Neurology 2003;60(7):1157–62.

96. Sicotte NL, Kern KC, Giesser BS, et al. Regional hippocampal atrophy in multiple sclerosis. Brain 2008;131(Pt 4):1134–41.

97. Wong EC, Buxton RB, Frank LR. Quantitative perfusion imaging using arterial spin labeling. Neuroimaging Clin N Am 1999;9(2):333–42.

98. Rashid W, Parkes LM, Ingle GT, et al. Abnormalities of cerebral perfusion in multiple sclerosis. J Neurol Neurosurg Psychiatr 2004;75(9):1288–93.

99. Wong EC, Luh WM, Liu TT, et al. Arterial spin labeling with higher SNR and temporal resolution. Magn Reson Med 2000;44(4):511–5.

100. Luh WM, Wong EC, Bandettini PA, et al. QUIPSS II with thin-slice TI1 periodic saturation: a method for improving accuracy of quantitative perfusion imaging using pulsed arterial spin labeling. Magn Reson Med 1999;41(6):1246–54.

101. Nestor PJ, Caine D, Fryer TD, et al. The topography of metabolic deficits in posterior cortical atrophy (the visual variant of Alzheimer's disease) with FDG-PET. J Neurol Neurosurg Psychiatry 2003;74(11):1521–9.

102. Matthews PM, Honey GD, Bullmore ET. Applications of fMRI in translational medicine and clinical practice. Nat Rev Neurosci 2006;7(9):732–44.

103. Lee M, Reddy H, Johansen-Berg H, et al. The motor cortex shows adaptive functional changes to brain injury from multiple sclerosis. Ann Neurol 2000;47(5):606–13.

104. Reddy H, Narayanan S, Matthews PM, et al. Relating axonal injury to functional recovery in MS. Neurology 2000;54(1):236–9.

105. Reddy H, Narayanan S, Arnoutelis R, et al. Evidence for adaptive functional changes in the cerebral cortex with axonal injury from multiple sclerosis. Brain 2000;123(Pt 11):2314–20.

106. Rocca MA, Colombo B, Falini A, et al. Cortical adaptation in patients with MS: a cross-sectional functional MRI study of disease phenotypes. Lancet Neurol 2005;4(10):618–26.

107. Mainero C, Caramia F, Pozzilli C, et al. fMRI evidence of brain reorganization during attention and memory tasks in multiple sclerosis. Neuroimage 2004;21(3):858–67.

108. Logothetis NK. What we can do and what we cannot do with fMRI. Nature 2008;453(7197):869–78.

109. Cifelli A, Matthews PM. Cerebral plasticity in multiple sclerosis: insights from fMRI. Mult Scler 2002;8(3):193–9.

110. Rocca MA, Filippi M. Functional MRI in multiple sclerosis. J Neuroimaging. 2007;17(Suppl 1):36S–41S.

111. Manson SC, Wegner C, Filippi M, et al. Impairment of movement-associated brain deactivation in multiple sclerosis: further evidence for a functional pathology of interhemispheric neuronal inhibition. Exp Brain Res 2008;187(1):25–31.

112. Manson SC, Palace J, Frank JA, et al. Loss of inter-hemispheric inhibition in patients with multiple sclerosis is related to corpus callosum atrophy. Exp Brain Res 2006;174(4):728–33.

113. Morgen K, Kadom N, Sawaki L, et al. Training-dependent plasticity in patients with multiple sclerosis. Brain 2004;127(Pt 11):2506–17.

114. Cader S, Cifelli A, Abu-Omar Y, et al. Reduced brain functional reserve and altered functional connectivity in patients with multiple sclerosis. Brain 2006;129(Pt 2):527–37.

115. Agosta F, Valsasina P, Caputo D, et al. Tactile-associated recruitment of the cervical cord is altered in patients with multiple sclerosis. Neuroimage 2008;39(4):1542–8.

116. Matthews PM, Johansen-Berg H, Reddy H. Non-invasive mapping of brain functions and brain recovery: applying lessons from cognitive neuroscience to neurorehabilitation. Restor Neurol Neurosci 2004;22(3–5):245–60.

117. Johansen-Berg H, Dawes H, Guy C, et al. Correlation between motor improvements and altered fMRI activity after rehabilitative therapy. Brain 2002;125(Pt 12):2731–42.

118. Buchli AD, Schwab ME. Inhibition of Nogo: a key strategy to increase regeneration, plasticity and functional recovery of the lesioned central nervous system. Annu Mediaev 2005;37(8):556–67.

119. Martino G. How the brain repairs itself: new therapeutic strategies in inflammatory and degenerative CNS disorders. Lancet Neurol 2004;3(6):372–8.

120. Saini S, DeStefano N, Smith S, et al. Altered cerebellar functional connectivity mediates potential adaptive plasticity in patients with multiple sclerosis. J Neurol Neurosurg Psychiatry 2004;75(6):840–6.

121. Rocca MA, Pagani E, Absinta M, et al. Altered functional and structural connectivities in patients with MS: a 3-T study. Neurology 2007;69(23):2136–45.

122. Wegner C, Filippi M, Korteweg T, et al. Relating functional changes during hand movement to clinical parameters in patients with multiple sclerosis in a multi-centre fMRI study. Eur J Neurol 2008;15(2):113–22.

123. Laule C, Vavasour IM, Kolind SH, et al. Magnetic resonance imaging of myelin. Neurotherapeutics 2007;4(3):460–84.

124. Laule C, Leung E, Lis DK, et al. Myelin water imaging in multiple sclerosis: quantitative correlations with histopathology. Mult Scler 2006;12(6): 747–53.

125. Laule C, Vavasour IM, Moore GR, et al. Water content and myelin water fraction in multiple sclerosis. A T2 relaxation study. J Neurol 2004;251(3): 284–93.

126. McGowan JC, Filippi M, Campi A, et al. Magnetisation transfer imaging: theory and application to multiple sclerosis. J Neurol Neurosurg Psychiatry 1998;64(Suppl 1):S66–9.

127. Chen JT, Collins DL, Atkins HL, et al. Magnetization transfer ratio evolution with demyelination and remyelination in multiple sclerosis lesions. Ann Neurol 2008;63(2):254–62.

128. Stankoff B, Wang Y, Bottlaender M, et al. Imaging of CNS myelin by positron-emission tomography. Proc Natl Acad Sci USA 2006;103(24):9304–9.

129. Herholz K. Cognitive dysfunction and emotional-behavioural changes in MS: the potential of positron emission tomography. J Neurol Sci 2006; 245(1–2):9–13.

130. Bakshi R, Miletich RS, Kinkel PR, et al. High-resolution fluorodeoxyglucose positron emission tomography shows both global and regional cerebral hypometabolism in multiple sclerosis. J Neuroimaging 1998;8(4):228–34.

131. Sorensen PS, Jonsson A, Mathiesen HK, et al. The relationship between MRI and PET changes and cognitive disturbances in MS. J Neurol Sci 2006; 245(1–2):99–102.

132. Blinkenberg M, Jensen CV, Holm S, et al. A longitudinal study of cerebral glucose metabolism, MRI, and disability in patients with MS. Neurology 1999;53(1):149–53.

133. Radu CG, Shu CJ, Shelly SM, et al. Positron emission tomography with computed tomography imaging of neuroinflammation in experimental autoimmune encephalomyelitis. Proc Natl Acad Sci U S A 2007;104(6):1937–42.

134. Venneti S, Lopresti BJ, Wiley CA. The peripheral benzodiazepine receptor (translocator protein 18kDa) in microglia: from pathology to imaging. Prog Neurobiol 2006;80(6):308–22.

135. Vowinckel E, Reutens D, Becher B, et al. PK11195 binding to the peripheral benzodiazepine receptor as a marker of microglia activation in multiple sclerosis and experimental autoimmune encephalomyelitis. J Neurosci Res 1997;50(2):345–53.

136. Banati RB, Newcombe J, Gunn RN, et al. The peripheral benzodiazepine binding site in the brain in multiple sclerosis: quantitative in vivo imaging of microglia as a measure of disease activity. Brain 2000;123(Pt 11):2321–37.

137. Vas A, Shchukin Y, Karrenbauer VD, et al. Functional neuroimaging in multiple sclerosis with radio-labelled glia markers: preliminary comparative PET studies with [11C]vinpocetine and [11C]PK11195 in patients. J Neurol Sci 2008;264(1–2):9–17.

138. Fujita M, Imaizumi M, Zoghbi SS, et al. Kinetic analysis in healthy humans of a novel positron emission tomography radioligand to image the peripheral benzodiazepine receptor, a potential biomarker for inflammation. Neuroimage 2008;40(1):43–52.

139. Evangelou N, Konz D, Esiri MM, et al. Size-selective neuronal changes in the anterior optic pathways suggest a differential susceptibility to injury in multiple sclerosis. Brain 2001;124(Pt 9): 1813–20.

140. Dutta R, McDonough J, Yin X, et al. Mitochondrial dysfunction as a cause of axonal degeneration in multiple sclerosis patients. Ann Neurol 2006; 59(3):478–89.

141. Lingford-Hughes A, Hume SP, Feeney A, et al. Imaging the GABA-benzodiazepine receptor subtype containing the alpha5-subunit in vivo with [11C]Ro15 4513 positron emission tomography. J Cereb Blood Flow Metab 2002;22(7):878–89.

142. Pike VW, Halldin C, Crouzel C, et al. Radioligands for PET studies of central benzodiazepine receptors and PK (peripheral benzodiazepine) binding sites—current status. Nucl Med Biol 1993;20(4):503–25.

143. Lendvai G, Velikyan I, Estrada S, et al. Biodistribution of 68Ga-labeled LNA-DNA mixmer antisense oligonucleotides for rat chromogranin-A. Oligonucleotides 2008;18(1):33–49.

144. Holt LJ, Herring C, Jespers LS, et al. Domain antibodies: proteins for therapy. Trends Biotechnol 2003;21(11):484–90.

High-Field Magnetic Resonance Imaging

Alayar Kangarlu, PhD

KEYWORDS

- High-field MR imaging • RF coils • High resolution
- MR spectroscopy • fMR imaging

Since its discovery, magnetic resonance (MR) has displayed capability for noninvasively transmitting information from the internal structures of opaque objects.[1,2] Introduction of gradients in the 1970s and its subsequent evolution into an imaging tool capable of revealing structure and function of biologic tissues has transformed MR imaging into an invaluable biomedical research method.[3,4] En route, clinical MR imaging operating at 1.5 T has also emerged as the most powerful modality for the study of the central nervous system (CNS). In addition to visualization of morphology, it has brought medicine other potentially powerful tools: functional MR imaging (fMR imaging),[5] spectroscopy (MRS),[6] and diffusion tensor (DT) MR imaging.[7] These tools have enabled MR imaging access to functional and microstructural aspects of the CNS.

Morphologic MR imaging enjoys a high signal-to-noise ratio (SNR) compared with other imaging modalities enabling it to acquire high-resolution images from the CNS.[8] The contrast-to-noise ratio (CNR) has been primarily governed by spin relaxation of spin-lattice (T1)–type and spin-spin (T2)–type; this has bestowed on MR imaging a high CNR for soft tissues.[9] MR imaging suffers from low pathologic specificity for many diseases. Integration of various MR modalities has been advanced as having the potential for enhancing specificity of MR imaging. The low SNR of some of these modalities (eg, MRS at 1.5 T) has prevented the potential of multimodality from being realized. At higher fields (4.0 T),[10–13] MR imaging has demonstrated ability to produce robust functional and spectroscopic data to achieve such integration of techniques under one protocol. It is known that the functional manifestations of a disease could possess genuine information in the presence of a normal structural image. The

same argument applies to the relationship between spectroscopic and morphologic images. As such, methods of improving quality of MR data are vigorously investigated.

This article explores the role of high-field (HF) MR imaging and ways that its advantages can best be used to unravel the secrets of diseases, such as multiple sclerosis (MS). Special emphasis is placed on morphologic imaging to highlight the role of soft tissue contrast, MRS to showcase ability of detecting biochemical information, and fMR imaging as an emerging technology for assessing tissue function with the possibility of eventual introduction to the clinical arena. In this context, HF indicates systems with a static magnetic field of 3.0 T or higher.

PHYSICS OF IMAGING

In all imaging techniques some form of wave, electromagnetic or sound, is used and the extent of absorption of individual atoms is manifested in an absorption or reflection map that makes up the image. A distinct aspect of these imaging methods is the characteristic time that interaction with matter takes (eg, of the order of nanoseconds in photography); these imaging techniques can produce images almost instantaneously. On the other hand, the interaction occurring between the electric field of the wave and the accelerating electrons of the subject attenuates the beam intensity, allowing an image to be formed. Because of the ability of electrons of the object to absorb the electric field oscillating at almost any frequency, the electric field strongly interacts with the tissue as it penetrates into the body. This characteristic of absorption imaging requires no preparation of the subjects, unlike MR imaging that uses

Columbia University College of Physicians and Surgeons and New York State Psychiatric Institute, 1051 Riverside Drive, New York, NY 10032, USA
E-mail address: ak2334@columbia.edu

Neuroimag Clin N Am 19 (2009) 113–128
doi:10.1016/j.nic.2008.09.008

radiofrequency (RF) waves that readily penetrate the biologic tissues. To achieve this, MR imaging requires a large magnet to "prime" the subject for RF absorption. On the other hand, the high energy of x-ray photons is capable of ionizing atoms and molecules while at the same time interacting strongly with the nucleus that limits the amount of waves that could be used for such imaging devices.

MR uses the magnetic field of electromagnetic waves in the RF range. RF waves have frequencies in MHz range (10^8 Hz), whereas x-rays have a frequency in AHz range (10^{18} Hz). Several physical quantities are involved in interaction of electromagnetic waves with matter, some of which are vectors and others are scalar quantities. In this section and throughout this article, vector quantities are designated by boldface and scalar quantities by regular fonts. Unlike electrons, which are monopoles, magnets require a dipole (ie, a magnetic dipole moment [μ]) with which to interact. This dipole is provided by the spinning action of the charged particles in atoms. Electrons and protons are charged particles and they spin. Spinning action assigns an angular momentum S to each particle. Interaction of the oscillating magnetic field (B_1) of an RF wave at a frequency of ω with a proton of μ magnetic moment is governed by the internal structure of the proton manifested in gyromagnetic ratio, γ, according to $\mu = \gamma S$. Clearly, on exposure of matter to a strong magnetic field (B_0), its protons will begin a presessional motion with a frequency known as Larmor frequency $\omega_L = \gamma B_0$. Resonance condition is produced when an RF coil is tuned such that its frequency $\omega = \omega_L$ enables its B_1 field to couple with precessing protons and transfer energy to them. The process is known as excitation. This narrow resonance condition is what imposes a stringent demand on the design and operation of RF coils. These coils can deliver a powerful RF pulse at resonance frequency ω_L to objects within a magnetic field (B_0) during the transmit path and absorb energy from the B_1 field of the protons during the receive path, which constitutes the MR imaging signal.

Absorption of RF causes protons to deflect away from the parallel direction with B_0, a process comparable to absorption of x-ray or light beam by atoms and molecules in CT and routine photography. The realignment of μ with B_0 is achieved through the mechanism of spin-lattice (T1) relaxation. T1-weighted images (T1W) produce one of the highest SNR sequences in MR imaging. Because T1 of various biologic tissues are of the order of 1 second, relaxation greatly slows down this imaging process. The need for repeated excitation of protons and detection of their emitted RF field while relaxing back to their equilibrium state makes a typical image with 256 × 256 pixels requiring roughly 256 seconds or about 4 minutes to acquire. Another important process in MR imaging is spin-spin relaxation or T2 decay. This process becomes significant because μ of individual atoms are not detectable at achievable B_0 in MR imaging scanners and that is why the sum of μ of a group of molecules within an imaginary box or voxel within the tissue is used. The net magnetic moment of this group is called magnetization vector or M. The magnitude of M depends on the extent of alignment of individual μ within the voxel. A maximum alignment is achieved in equilibrium and immediately after delivery of an RF pulse at ω_L. Because of local inhomogeneities in B_0, however, coherent precession of M about B_0 is lost over time. This loss of alignment occurs at a rate known as spin-spin relaxation or T2. T2-weighted (T2W) images in MR imaging are rich with information about local structures. The use of T1W images is another way that MR imaging can produce brain maps with distinct contrast between various tissues, which is clinically useful in MS. Many other useful contrast mechanisms are offered by MR imaging, which may be sensitive to many aspects of CNS pathology of MS. This multiple means of accessing biologic tissues during the same session makes MR imaging the ideal technique with multimodal approach to the study of a disease.

HIGH-FIELD MR IMAGING

Soon after the appearance of MR imaging scanners for medical applications, 1.5 T was recognized as the high field strength for clinical scanners. This field strength was later accepted as the standard clinical field for MR imaging scanners. Nevertheless, efforts by researchers to test the advantages and viabilities of higher fields began right away.[11,12] Research scanners have always shadowed the clinical scanners keeping research field strengths higher than their clinical counterparts. During the 1980s and early 1990s, when the standard clinical filed was 1.5 T, the B_0 of research scanners stood at 3.0 T and 4.0 T.[11-13] Despite their limited numbers, the researchers using 4.0 T whole-body scanners worked on many important issues, such as feasibility of imaging at HF, safety, RF coil and gradient design, and pulse sequence development, which paved the road for the development of 3.0 T scanners by major manufacturers for clinical uses.

A similar history is now unfolding for higher fields. An 8.0 T[14] whole-body scanner was developed in the mid-1990s, which was followed by manufacturers' development of whole-body 7.0 T scanners of today. At present, some 20 institutions around the world have received commercial 7.0 T MR imaging scanners and another 30 will be in possession of these devices within the next 5 years, raising their total to around 50. This trend is remarkable considering that only a handful of 4.0 T scanners were built in the late 1980s and 1990s as a precursor to today's clinical 3.0 T scanners.[11–13] A flurry of HF technology development has erupted in which, for a large part, efforts have been focused on the understanding of problems of MR imaging at high fields. These researchers have produced many innovative solutions to many challenges of HF imaging. These challenges include magnet design, safety, RF coils, artifacts, slow imaging process, and so forth. The understanding of these issues will help appreciation of their role in the progress of this field and will contribute to the incorporation of HF MR imaging in biomedical research.

THE MAGNET

Some difficult constraints have to be incorporated in the design of magnets for human applications, primarily because of the need to contain the human body within the scanner. Cylindrical wire wounds or solenoids have been shown to have solutions for Laplace equation $\nabla^2 B_Z = 0$, which has spherical harmonics as its solution in the form of terms called Legendre polynomials. Solutions of equation with spherical symmetry determine magnetic field components due to each current loop in the central regions of the magnet. Generation of axial magnetic field at the center of the magnet at the space required to image major human organs places constraints on the size of the magnets.[15] The central region is called diameter spherical volume (DSV) and is about 50 cm, allowing images of regions as large as the human abdominal section within the scanner. It is conceivable that magnets with fields even higher than 9.4 T, which is currently the highest field for human MR imaging, will be designed and built in the future. HF magnets appropriate for MR imaging built as solenoids of superconducting wires capable of carrying hundreds of amperes are likely to be designed with alloys capable of currying higher currents or more wires wound around the former. NbTi is the alloy used in almost all magnets built for biomedical applications with field strength of up to 10 T, because of the current density that these wires can carry within their own magnetic fields. This phenomenon makes fields greater than 10 T difficult to attain for whole-body magnets of NbTi because the reduced current density in the wires requires the use of massive amounts of superconducting wires that makes such designs

unfeasible. These magnets should operate at less than NbTi critical temperature, Tc = 10 K, making 4.2 K, the boiling temperature of liquid helium (LHe2), appropriate for sustained NbTi superconductivity. To achieve higher fields, one could pump on LHe2 to drive the temperature to 1.8 K, which is the triple point of LHe2; this allows fields of up to 15 T to be attained with this technology. Another approach would be the use of NbSb, which can produce fields of up to 15 T at 4.2 K. One consequence of present technology is the massive size and weight of the scanners. All present HF MR imaging whole-body scanners use NbTi; they weigh up to 30 tons and contain up to 80 MJ of energy. The magnets are about 3 m long and equally high. Their shielding would add to their weight and size. The cryogenic technology of closed-cycle refrigeration has greatly helped the use of LHe2 consumption for these magnets. The LHe2 boil-off rate of early HF magnets was high, as much as 10 L per day. At present, there are zero–boil off 7.0 T scanners with physical characteristics comparable to those of early generations. For unshielded magnets, 5 Gauss line of the stray field extends to about 10 m axially depending on the bore diameter. The weight of the magnets is roughly 4 ton/T. One way of containing the stray field of the unshielded HF systems is passive shielding that consists of an iron room being built around the magnet. Such B_0 shields could bring the 5 Gauss line to within 2 m of the magnet depending on the amount of steel used to build the shield. For 7.0 T magnets, a B_0 shield of 300 to 400 ton iron will suffice to bring the stray field to within close distances of the magnet. The cost of building such a B_0 shield room is about $500 thousand plus or minus $200 thousand, depending on the location and management of the shield room design and construction.

SAFETY

The strong static magnetic field used in MR imaging can pose some safety and health hazards to human subjects. These can be divided into three main categories: missile or projectile effect, magnetohydrodynamic (MHD), and RF power deposition.[16,17]

The missile effect refers to the magnetization of any ferromagnetic material in the near vicinity of magnets. In general, an object with a magnetization vector of **M** will experience a rotational force or torque of $\tau = \mathbf{M} \times \mathbf{B}$, which will force **M** to line up with **B**, here B_0. This force is the same one that lines up the compass needle with the magnetic field of the earth and lines up the molecular dipole moments μ of water with B_0 in the human body within MR imaging scanners. This torque can be strong enough to cause displacement of medical devices implanted in the human body. Medical devices are usually tested for the values of torque acting on them if they contain ferromagnetic or strongly paramagnetic components. Recently, many medical devices are being tested within the highest field strengths available for human imaging (ie, 7.0 T and higher)[18] to demonstrate their safety. In addition, the presence of static magnetic field inhomogeneity (∇B_0) gives rise to a translational force of $F=\nabla(\tau)$, which makes the magnitude of **F** proportional to the product of **B** and spatial variations of magnetic field $\partial\mathbf{B}/\partial z$. This force is of attractive nature and additionally is proportional to the magnetic susceptibility χ of the object within the field. For HF magnets, given that these magnets have a high B_0 inhomogeneity ($\partial B/\partial z$) near the opening of the magnet, the high B_0 will result in a high $B_0\partial B_0/\partial z$, which is about 40 T^2/m. If ferromagnetic objects with high χ are introduced into this region of high $B_0\partial B_0/\partial z$, they experience a large attractive force that pulls them toward the center of the scanner. This force, untamed, could turn any ferrous metals brought into the scanner room into a missile zeroed in on its target—the center of the magnet. The impact of such fast-moving objects poses a lethal threat to any living being within the magnet. The missile effect constitutes the most ominous preventable risk for operation of HF magnets.

Another venue for expression of such translational force is the blood within the vessels, the MHD. The high conductivity of blood causes its flow to generate a force due to the B_0 acting on the blood moving in a perpendicular direction to the field. This force generates an electric current normal to the axis of vessels which, in turn, interacts with the magnetic field to generate a force against the blood flow, hence lowering the blood pressure. In the past, it had been estimated that at 10 T a large increase in blood pressure of more than 20% would be needed to neutralize this MHD force to maintain the flow in the aorta.[19] This phenomenon is highly directional and its effect may be averaged out as a result of the randomness of blood vessel directions that causes the blood within them to experience a randomly directed force; this could be one of the reasons that no such change in blood pressure has been observed in studies on animals within HF magnets.[17,20]

Characteristics of RF waves required for excitation of spins in MR imaging is also a matter of safety. In general, the interaction of electromagnetic waves with objects depends on the relative value of their wavelength, λ, to the dimension of the object, d. As the field strength increases, the proton's Larmor frequency (f) increases causing λ to decrease proportionally as a consequence of the relationship f = c/λ, where c is the speed of light. Furthermore, the wavelength of RF drops according to $\lambda_b=\lambda/\sqrt{\varepsilon}$ as it penetrates into the body with a permittivity of ε. Consequently, the in-tissue wavelength or λ_b drops rapidly as B_0 increases. At 7.0 T, where λ = 1 m, the RF penetration into a water phantom will reduce the wavelength to about 11 cm because of the ε of water being around 80. Considering the typical dimension of the human head being around d = 15 cm, at 7.0 T λ_b < d, a condition that reveals the wave nature of the RF in its propagation through the medium. This condition establishes a strong inhomogeneity in RF amplitude as it spreads through the medium. Such RF inhomogeneity, in high dielectric media, such as water or human head as shown in **Fig. 1**, creates a condition for concentration or focusing of RF waves in a central region. Although the extent of this dielectric resonance is relatively large, it warrants mentioning a condition known as "hot spots" that can pose a health risk to subjects in the extreme case of highly inhomogeneous RF distribution of coils at HF. In this case, efforts must be made to achieve the most homogeneous RF fields possible. It must be noted that although such homogeneous fields are necessary for safe operation of MR imaging scanners at ultra HF, the desirable level of homogeneity might not be achievable with simple designs of RF coils. In addition to safety considerations, RF homogeneity is also essential for uniform imaging. Recent developments in parallel imaging have made much progress in providing uniform RF distribution and elimination of RF focusing at HF. For HF scanners, transmitting surface coils and other specialty coils still could potentially pose a safety concern

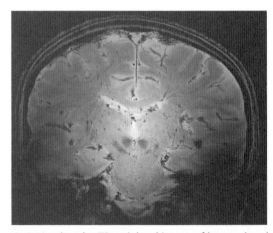

Fig. 1. A spin echo T2-weighted image of human head acquired at 8.0 T. The image parameters were TR = 750 milliseconds, TE = 25 milliseconds, matrix = 1024 × 1024.

because they could produce highly nonuniform RF fields. Significance of knowledge of localized heating is that physiologic facility for heat removal from a highly localized internal region is poor, unlike the body's ability to dissipate heat from superficial tissues. Furthermore, regulatory guidelines for maximum RF exposures usually do not take into account the possibility of localized heating because this is a characteristic of RF coil design and operation. Although one could be within the regulatory limits for RF power application on a human subject, an inhomogeneous RF distribution could still create a potentially hazardous condition for localized internal tissue heating.

SIGNAL-TO-NOISE RATIO AND CONTRAST-TO-NOISE RATIO

The factors affecting SNR are B_0, RF coil design, pulse sequence parameters, number of averages, voxel size, gradient strength of phase encoding, and receiver bandwidth. From these factors, all but B_0 are changeable after the scanner is purchased. Assuming that all other factors are optimized, therefore, B_0 becomes the sole determinant of SNR.

A static magnetic field of the order of greater than 0.1 T is required to generate images from the magnetic dipoles of atoms and molecules of the human body. Exposure of tissue water to a $B_0 = 1.0$ T will split the spin population into parallel (−) and antiparallel (+) in orientation with $\mathbf{B_0}$. The difference in energy level of $E_+ - E_- = \Delta E = 2\mu.\mathbf{B_0}$ will develop as a result of interaction of μ with $\mathbf{B_0}$. At 1.0 T, this energy difference is about 10^{-7} eV or 0.1 μeV. This number should be compared with the atomic energy levels of the order of 1eV and room temperature energy of about 25 meV. In this highly unfavorable environment for detection of MR signal, the resonance coupling of the RF coil with precessing protons drastically reduces the noise spectrum enabling the detection of such feeble signal from the background noise. As the excess population of parallel protons, (ie, the ratio of $E_+/E_- \sim e(-\Delta E/kT)$) increases, it results in a twofold advantage for detection of their signal. First, it increases the energy gap or $\Delta E/kT$, which means that there is larger population of RF photons. Second, the RF wave or RF photon energies are higher. Both of these effects contribute to higher SNR as B_0 increases. This SNR advantage highlights the role of high magnetic fields in MR imaging.

In the case of 7.0 T scanners, SNR is about five times higher than at 1.5 T. Compared with the typical voxel size at 1.5 T (ie, 1 mm × 1 mm × 5 mm) the SNR at HF indicates that signal from a single voxel is approaching the limits of biologic cells

(ie, 10–100 μm). In approaching microscopic detection capability, the role of relaxation rates should also be taken into account. They represent the time scale during which the MR signal persists after it is generated. Although T1 is of the order of 1 second, T2 is almost 10 times shorter for biologic tissues. In addition, relaxation rates are B_0 dependent. T2 decreases while T1 increases with B_0. At 7.0 T, in vivo T1 values reported for gray matter (GM) are around 2 seconds and those for white matter (WM) are about 1.3 seconds; T1 values at 3.0 T for GM are around 1.5 seconds and those for WM are about 0.8 seconds; and T1 at 1.5 T for GM is around 1.2 seconds and those for WM are about 0.6 seconds.[21] Based on these values, GM/WM contrast at 1.5 T is 0.67, at 3.0 T is 0.69, and at 7.0 T is 0.42. In this method of calculation of contrast, the difference in SNR between GM and WM is divided by their average values. The magnitude of GM/WM contrast or CNR is clearly on a down trend as B_0 increases beyond 7.0 T, but not by much. T1 values often depend on the techniques used for their measurements, however. Nevertheless, converging of T1 values has been expected as B_0 increases. T2 relaxations are also monitored for their B_0 dependence. At 7.0 T, T2 values reported for GM are around 55 milliseconds, whereas those for WM are about 46 milliseconds. T2 values at 3.0 T for GM are around 110 milliseconds and for WM are about 80 milliseconds; at 1.5 T these values are around 93 milliseconds for GM and 76 milliseconds for WM.[21-23] Based on these values, GM/WM contrast at 1.5 T is 0.32, at 3.0 T is 0.32, and at 7.0 T is 0.18. In these measurements, the in-plane resolution has been kept at nearly 1 mm.

Relaxation measurements are also used to produce the so-called "relaxometry maps." They provide valuable knowledge on the whole brain containing information on the microscopic structure of the brain. Relaxometry requires long acquisition times and that is why it has not been widely used in the clinical settings. Some techniques have been recently developed to accelerate their measurements and, as a consequence, to avail their benefits to the studies of neurodevelopment and diseases.[24] At HF, high-resolution relaxation measurements enable MR to visualize very small structures in brain regions as voxel dimensions approache scales of microvessels and eventually individual cells.[25] Gradient echo (GRE) images taken at HF reveal vast microvascular networks networks, as shown in **Fig. 2**, which have never been seen before at lower fields. GRE is used for T2* measurements, whereas spin echo (SE) is required for T1 and T2 measurements. Recent measurements at 3.0 T using fast SE (FSE) have shown

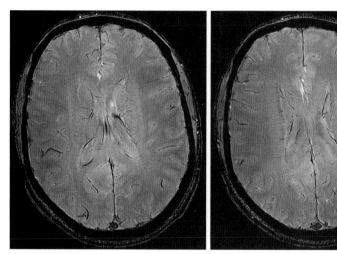

Fig. 2. Susceptibility-weighted images acquired at 7.0 T in the axial plane, demonstrating exquisite details of the blood vessels with respect to which any possible abnormality could be identified. Image was acquired on a Philips Achieva 7.0 T. (*Courtesy of* Philips Medical Systems, Cleveland, Ohio, USA; with permission.)

interesting patterns of T1 and T2 changes in brain tissues.[24] As the SNR increases, relaxometry becomes more practical at 7.0 T and higher, which will provide valuable information about normal brain development. Similar work on disease progression would offer information about different mechanisms affecting the decay of transverse magnetization, which better characterizes the constituents of the voxel. This way, processes at the molecular level will translate into information that will enhance MR imaging specificity for the study of various diseases.

High resolution is one way of using the SNR currency at HF. As resolution increases, the number of protons (signal), noise spectrum, and contribution from partial volume effects decrease. Voxels contain the source of MR signal (ie, protons) and the source of noise (ie, everything else). Noise is also caused by several B_0-independent mechanisms that are distinct from that generating the signal. These mechanisms include: (a) random fluctuation of μ, (b) thermal noise from the circuitry of the RF coil, (c) physiologic noise, and (d) and receiver bandwidth. Fluctuation of μ giving rise to nuclear spin noise spectra has been predicted theoretically and measured experimentally.[26] Thermal noise is governed by (a) random electromagnetic signal generated in the body due to the movement of ions and other charged particles, (b) electronics noise generated by RF amplifiers, transmit and receive electronics, and RF coil structure, and (c) the receiver bandwidth. At HF, most of these contributions remain comparable to those of low-field MR imaging or increase linearly with B_0. MR signal increases quadratically with B_0.[27–30] Increase in

SNR is therefore in large part generated by increase in signal strength, which is caused by high B_0. In addition to SNR, CNR determines the information content of MR images. Higher SNR and CNR are ideal for visualization of brain anatomy and pathophysiology. Although SNR is almost linearly dependent on B_0, field dependence of CNR is more complicated. Resolution and CNR are the quantities that must be optimized by the choice of proper pulse sequence parameters. The high-resolution images in **Fig. 3** show a comparison of 3.0 T and 7.0 T whole-brain acquisition. Although the higher resolution of 7.0 T represents the higher SNR, there is a distinct difference in WM/GM contrast between the two images. Experimental quantification of SNR and CNR with equivalent parameters corrected for field strength will elucidate the actual gain in HF compared to lower field strengths.

The gain in inherent SNR in MR is established as a function of magnetic field. The actual increase in SNR varies as a function of many factors, however, including sequence parameters and hardware. For clinical MR imaging, the present consensus is that 3.0 T scanners hold a twofold advantage over 1.5 T systems (see **Fig. 3**). Similarly, scanning at 7.0 T compared with 3.0 T could further double the SNR. High-resolution in vivo images of humans have been acquired at 100 μm in-plane resolution at the turn of the millennium.[25] For the first time, ability to reduce the voxels of MR imaging images down to 20 nL demonstrated the ability of MR imaging to visualize exquisite details of human neuroanatomy. Images acquired under similar acquisition conditions have at least twice the SNR and much better

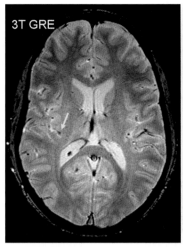 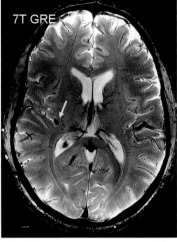

Fig. 3. Gradient echo images acquired at 3.0 T and 7.0 T. (*Courtesy of* Dr. Yulin Ge, New York University, NY, USA.)

representation of details and microstructures, including the WM fibers and GM microscopic blood vessels. Higher SNR advantages of HF MR imaging could be used to reduce the voxel size to achieve higher resolution or shorter repetition time (TR), echo time (TE), and readout time, which, in turn, leads to faster acquisition. Both of these advantages are valuable in the clinical setting.

The use of high SNR for higher resolution has many advantages. As voxels approach microscopic range, the population of water molecules confined within the voxel decreases. Assuming that incorporation of recent technologies, such as parallel imaging, will further increase the SNR, it is conceivable that a factor of 10 reduction in voxel volume of HF images compared with clinical MR imaging is within reach. Already, 100^3 μm^3 images have been acquired from murine and rhesus monkey at HF range. MR imaging at 9.4 T has been shown to reveal cytoarchitecture of the human cerebral cortex of excised brain tissues.[31] Typically, HF images have good GM/WM contrast over the entire brain. In addition to such exquisite details in cortical imaging, subcortical regions reveal high MR imaging contrast, which allows microscopic demarcation of anatomic structures, such as the basal ganglia. Significance of basal ganglia is that it is the locus of a collection of nuclei that affect descending motor pathways and cognition and emotion. Damages to the basal ganglia in MS can be associated with several symptoms. The ability to correlate symptoms, such as involuntary movements, tremor, weakness, and spasticity, with high-resolution images of basal ganglia may be useful in managing patients who have MS. Also, the ability of an accurate delineation of basal ganglia plays an important role in studies of dementia, addiction, and psychiatric diseases.

Contrast at HF is highly affected by iron particles due to tissue ferritin. These iron particles add to the endogenous T2 contrast in the brain resulting in lower T2 in the brain nuclei. This hypointensity increases with B_0. The distinct contrast in the basal ganglia and the dentate nucleus of the cerebellum at HF are shown to correlate to high iron concentration as measured by postmortem histology.[32] It is becoming clear now that as B_0 increases from 1.5 T to 3.0 T, ability to use thin slices combined with extra paramagnetic contrast reveals a large number of small brain nuclei and cortical regions.

The shortened T2 enhances the visibility of these nuclei compared with surrounding regions, a feature that has many clinical applications because of the possibility of its rapid acquisition. As B_0 increases toward 7.0 T, many brain nuclei, such as caudate nucleus and globus pallidus, gain even higher T2 contrast (see **Fig. 1**). In addition to spin-spin relaxation, smaller voxel size, which implies a higher sensitivity to diffusion, makes it possible to have a more significant contribution to T2 contrast at HF. It is believed that MR imaging is capable of offering information on subvoxel levels. DT MR imaging is one such method that uses the sensitivity of MR signal to water diffusion to reveal order in biologic tissues. Although DT MR imaging fiber tracking is gaining more acceptance as still another promising diagnostic tool, more molecular information could be gained from HF MR images because they contain more information from the tissue structure at the molecular level. MR can indeed give insight into molecular and cellular structures of tissues using some processes (eg, diffusion and perfusion). Both diffusion and perfusion are fundamentally important to the viability of biologic tissues and they are present in all of them. The use of diffusion mechanism makes dimensions smaller than those of the voxel accessible to imaging by MR. As SNR increases to enable submillimeter voxels to shrink further toward microscopic dimensions diffusion has to become more prominent in determining contrast in sequences not even sensitized for diffusion detection, such as routine SE and GRE. For these practical reasons, HF has potential for fascinating and challenging opportunities to study the human brain for structural and functional information never accessible before. HF MR imaging could revolutionize clinical practice, because of the enormous power in probing molecular events giving it flexibility and versatility that all other imaging techniques lack. Events at the molecular and cellular levels will become more important at HF MR and once sequences are optimized to incorporate their effect in the overall image contrast, many more techniques will be able to detect subvoxel structures and functions as DT MR imaging and high-resolution fMR imaging do now.

MR imaging soft tissue contrast is further empowered by high resolution at HF. As resolution increases and voxel volume decreases, susceptibility-based signal dropouts become more significant. Such susceptibility is either due to tissue inhomogeneity or the presence of paramagnetic elements, such as iron; this greatly enhances the contrast between the brain parenchyma and blood vessels making even microscopic vessels more visible,[33–35] which is ideal for brain tumor diagnosis and therapy monitoring. Achieving such resolution at lower fields is difficult because they both lack the required susceptibility contrast and require long acquisition times, which are not clinically feasible.

Considering the converging of relaxations, work has already begun to enhance the contrast of HF images. One such method is susceptibility based and it improves the tissue conspicuity by phase contrast.[36] At 7.0 T, images have been acquired with voxels in less than 100 nL with a strong phase contrast,[34] which is capable of enhancing the contrast between and within GM and WM. CNR between GM and WM on GRE phase images from normal volunteers with about 60 nL resolution have been acquired ranging from 3 to 20 over the cortex, which amounts to a drastic increase in CNR, an almost 10-fold advantage compared to non–phase-enhanced techniques. Adding multichannel detection advantage to phase sensitivity could increase CNR by another order of magnitude. The underlying mechanism for phase enhancement is magnetic susceptibility—both endogenous and exogenous. Iron plays an important role in microvascular-laden GM tissues. In GM, this adds

contrast to images of this tissue, which allows the layering of GM to be revealed. Such high contrast is because at HF, in addition to difference in tissue density, images are sensitive to structural differences, such as vascularity between the layers. Enhanced CNR in WM might be associated with the size of fiber bundles. Lower vascular density within WM has made it look homogeneous on lower-field images but at HF fiber bundles seem to generate enough difference in magnetic susceptibility to create intra-WM contrast (see **Fig. 1**). MS diagnostics and distinction between various lesions in different WM locations may benefit from such intra-WM contrast. Phase contrast sequences at lower fields were primarily used in MR angiography because the change in the phase shifts only due to flowing water molecules could produce phase change high enough to distinguish vessels from the surrounding stationary tissues. HF is now offering phase images that generate contrast between adjacent stationery spins. At HF, therefore, magnetic field gradients are generated as a result of normal structural variations in similar tissue constituents. Such capability has already been used in enhancing the contrast between normal tissues and lesions and to generate contrast to reveal details of what is known as normal-appearing WM.[37] This aspect of HF MR imaging has more untapped potential for further improvement in intra-tissue contrast enhancements. This potential warrants a better understanding of the role of susceptibility at HF.

MAGNETIC SUSCEPTIBILITY

Magnetic susceptibility, χ, represents the extent to which matter magnetizes when placed in a strong magnetic field. It is useful at this point to review the notion of magnetic field (**H**), magnetic induction (**B**), and magnetization (**M**). **M** refers to the total magnetic moments per unit volume $\mathbf{M} = \sum \mu/v$. **M** is caused by **H** according to $\mathbf{M} = \chi\mathbf{H}$. **B** and **H** are also related by the expression $\mathbf{B} = \mu_0\mathbf{H}$, where μ_0 is the permittivity of free space and is $4\pi \times 10^{-7}$ Henry/m. The units of **B** and **H** in SI unit system are T and A/m, respectively. Magnetic field intensity inside an object with magnetization **M** is $\mathbf{B} = \mu_0(\mathbf{M} + \mathbf{H})$. Substitution of expression for **M** makes $\mathbf{B} = \mu\mathbf{H}$, where $\mu = \mu_0(1 + \chi)$ is the magnetic permeability of matter. The entire information about susceptibility of an object and how it is related to the **B,** or **B$_0$** as it is called in MR imaging, is lumped into μ through χ. Modulation of **B$_0$** by χ, the so-called "susceptibility effect," causes a mechanism of contrast between tissues that is **B$_0$** dependent. If difference in susceptibility, $\Delta\chi$, between adjacent tissues is small (eg, of the order of B_0 inhomogeneity) such contrast could be used for better visualization of tissues, such as blood vessels. Very high $\Delta\chi$, as at the air/tissue interfaces, causes large signal dropouts interfering with studies focused on these regions. For instance, fMR imaging studies of dorsolateral prefrontal cortex fall into this category.

As for advantages of susceptibility, it is easy to see that **M** within a voxel is directly proportional to B_0 making HF ideal for susceptibility-based enhancements. T2* effects will enhance proportional to the magnetic field. As seen in **Fig. 4** an exquisite contrast is obtained on these images taken at 7.0 T. Considering the high T2* decay rate due to paramagnetic susceptibility of deoxyhemoglobin, these structures will have their dimensions exaggerated resulting in better visualization of vasculature network in the brain as it is clear in **Fig. 4**. In vivo vascular imaging could be used in establishing a relationship between brain tumor vascularization and functional imaging results, vascular disorders, brain development, brain tumor staging, and MS. In the case of MS, lack of specificity of imaging modalities has contributed to the persistence of diagnostic work-up based on multiple criteria. Despite its unsurpassed ability in visualizing lesions, MR imaging has yet to be established as a reliable tool for diagnosis of MS or any other diseases. A reliable assessment of the cerebral microvascular system may go a long way to increase the role of MR imaging in the diagnosis of MS. This issue is distinct from SNR in which ancillary technologies, such as multichannel detection, could improve the existing situation. In other words, no matter how much we succeed in improving the SNR of 3.0 T, because of the absence of B_0-dependent susceptibility contrast, its microvascular depiction will never match those of 7.0 T magnets.

RADIOFREQUENCY AND GRADIENT COIL TECHNOLOGY

RF coil technology has experienced many advances for adaptation to HF. The traditional bird-cage designs have proved unable to address all HF challenges. Transverse electromagnetic coils have been shown to be able to more readily lend themselves to tuning and matching at frequencies of 300 MHz and higher. Both designs reveal highly inhomogeneous images at HF, however (see **Fig. 1**). Concerns for excessive heat deposition predicted by B_0^2-dependence of RF power was highlighted as the first images at 8.0 T were acquired.[38,39] Dielectric effects showed to be able to focus RF power at the central regions of the head. This effect caused inhomogeneous spread of RF over the head reducing power required in the peripheral regions for spin excitation. Furthermore, there are two primary methods for acceleration of image acquisition based on parallel imaging: SMASH-like methods and SENSE-like methods.[40,41] Both methods use each coil element to provide information that helps with the reconstruction of under-sampled images. In fact, in both techniques, RF encoding partially replaces gradient encoding. In SMASH, the k-space is reconstructed using signal from different coil elements to act as spatial harmonics that should have been generated by phase-encoding (PE) gradients. These harmonics perform the retrospective encoding that would have been done by PE

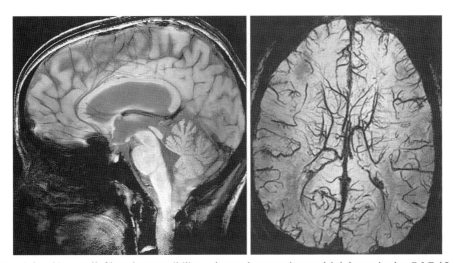

Fig. 4. T2* weighted image (*left*) and susceptibility-enhanced venous image (*right*) acquired at 7.0 T. (*Courtesy of* Prof. John Gore, Vanderbilt University.)

gradients, which amounts to shifting the k-space. Parallel transmit restores RF distribution over the entire head and directly addresses the SAR concerns. Combination multichannel receive and transmit technology will help HF to obtain anatomic MR images with microscopic resolution, blood oxygen level dependent (BOLD) and perfusion-based images with high temporal and spatial resolutions, high-resolution fiber tracking, and metabolite maps of glutamate and γ-aminobutyric acid (GABA), the most important excitatory and inhibitory neurotransmitters in the human brain. In addition to in vivo studies, HF scanners are a powerful tool to noninvasively investigate a wide range of biologic processes in isolated perfused organs, single cells, tissues ex vivo, and protein solutions. Furthermore, positron emission tomography (PET), which is another powerful tool for probing physiologic events at the cellular level, is extensively used by many investigators to study the brain. Because of the complementary nature of microPET and MR imaging, equipped with new RF multichannel transmit/receive technology could also be used for serial MR/PET studies combining metabolic, anatomic, and physiologic information of MR imaging with that of PET for a more comprehensive exploration of any phenomena in the same experiment.

Development of more powerful diagnostic imaging has also been helped by availability of more robust gradients. Although in the past most clinical scanners were equipped with gradients with strength of 20 mT/m and slew rate of 50 T/m/sec, the role of stronger gradients in HF has encouraged work in this area, resulting in more powerful gradient designs. Most of the efforts in echo planar imaging (EPI) research have been directed toward minimizing image artifacts. These advances are in gradient coil design and gradient amplifiers. Also, active shielding (AS) of gradients has become a viable option. AS drastically reduces the eddy currents and their harmful artifacts. Better pre-emphasis and improved gradient amplifiers also have contributed in making modern gradients more versatile. HF gradients typically have strengths of 50 to 100 mT/m and they can switch on and off in 150 to 300 microseconds; this increases the slew rate up to 200 to 500 T/m/s. Strong gradients with shorter switching times are particularly useful for recovering signal losses and suppressing T2* artifacts. The dB/dt of switching gradients will induce electric fields that can cause nerve stimulation. This gradient-induced electric field could be high enough to induce ventricular fibrillation if dB/dt is not limited. The safe operations of gradients are secured by regulatory agencies to ensure that induced electric fields in the body are kept far below uncomfortable

levels. One way of using high gradient while avoiding its undesirable aspects is the use of asymmetric gradients, which only apply their field over the intended body part (ie, the head) to keep the heart isolated from induced electric fields. Head-only HF scanners are in operation today in many centers. HF does not necessarily imply the use of higher gradient strength or slew rate to obtain high resolution images, because higher SNR at HF is caused by increased excess protons in each voxel providing higher in-plane resolution. Stronger gradients must be eventually used to achieve isotropic voxels, however. Stronger gradients are beneficial to achieve high resolution in the frequency and phase-encoding directions also. They are also important in determining the resolution and scanning times. High gradient strengths and short rise times are particularly desirable for EPI. Because fMR imaging is one of the primary beneficiaries of HF, many HF scanners are designed with more robust gradients and while clinical scanners are limited to less than 50 mT/m, the smaller bore gradient coils used for asymmetric gradients on research systems used up to 100 mT/m and animal scanners are designed for up to 1000 mT/m.

STRUCTURAL IMAGING

Morphologic images with high resolution are invaluable in the study of structural changes caused by diseases. High-resolution images are important because they contain more details of the microstructures. Furthermore, high-resolution images are less vulnerable to partial volume averaging, because voxel sizes are approaching the smaller unit cell sizes forming the tissues. Volumetric measurements of selected brain structures are routinely performed in research labs. They are carried out using T1W three-dimensional acquisitions that can be reformatted to generate images along the planes of interest to most clearly visualize the regions of interest (ROI). Neuroscientists conduct a large number of volumetric studies involving delineation of various brain ROIs in many brain diseases. Accuracy of these volumetric measurements is a function of precision in defining tissue boundaries. HF MR imaging greatly enhances this precision as boundaries are better defined because of smaller voxels and lower partial volume effects.

At 7.0 T and higher, such volumetric studies could be carried out with microscopic resolution. Alternatively, the high SNR could be used to achieve faster imaging to suppress some physiologic motions. These physiologic motions (ie, respiratory motion, heart beat, brain cerebrospinal fluid pulsatile motion, and so forth) strongly affect the resolution of in vivo imaging. A field strength of 7.0 T is appropriate for in vivo MR imaging to produce images revealing microscopic details (see **Figs. 1–3**). The stronger gradients and powerful RF pulses of HF scanners combined with other progress in MR technology, such as parallel imaging,[40,41] is presently capable of drastically reducing the acquisition time up to a factor of five. In fact, with whole-body scanners operating at 11.7 T, the in vivo acquisition of a whole-brain image with isotropic 100-μm resolution enabling study of focal morphology, pathophysiology, and its functional consequences in brain diseases, will soon be within reach.

In addition, at HF both T1W and T2W images could be modified to measure T1 and T2 values over the entire brain or locally with high resolution. In particular, T2W images in which the contrast is generated by the T2 of the water protons with a sensitive dependence on the mobility of the water molecules could provide T2 maps over the entire brain. This process is of great value in diagnosis of pathology because any damage on the brain causes an increase in T2 value of that region. This focal increase in T2 is generated as a result of loss of the tight organization of the brain resulting in an increase of T2 that can be measured by MR imaging. High-resolution T2 relaxometry is a powerful technique based on systematic acquisition of T2W images at different TEs that allow computation of T2 values over the whole brain. The focal values of T2 offer a highly sensitive and objective means for identification of abnormal structures and function.[42] Although T2 relaxometry has been used for the identification of hippocampal[43] and amygdala abnormalities,[44] our lab is presently conducting studies in which T2 relaxometry is used on the study of infant brain development at 3.0 T with an eight-channel receive technology. Multichannel technology has great potential for making significant improvement on the T2 values acquired from human subjects in 3.0 T studies compared to 1.5 T studies. Similar work for T1 and T2 values could be conducted on the 7.0 T systems with an immensely valuable gain of information. Furthermore, parallel imaging lends itself more readily to HF applications, owing to the highly localized nature of field-of-view (FOV) of individual coil elements and this inherent RF inhomogeneity can be incorporated well in acquiring unique images from the same subject. Undersampled images of parallel receivers have to be unfolded. Suppression of the inhomogeneity depends on a well-designed unfolding routine, which is ameliorated by the limited penetration depth at HF. Multichannel receivers will make the best use of the high SNR at HF. Design of highly

parallel coils will undoubtedly further enhance HF for wider applications. Combination of HF and additional sensitivity of multichannel RF coils will enhance the chances of detecting subtle effects, such as distinction of new lesions in MS from old ones, in vivo grading of brain tumor, and relaxation changes during early brain development. The ability to build multichannel RF coils with more channels will provide an additional source of enhancement of image qualities. Very high resolution images could be acquired in shorter time from a 7.0 T scanner. The detection of some details of the human brain, such as the sharp GM/WM boundary and trilaminar structure of the cortex, is a clear indication of the compound benefits of all the aforementioned effects. Such images enable study of morphologic manifestation of diseases at an unprecedented clarity and resolution, which will provide investigators with a powerful tool with which they could explore their scientific hypotheses.

HIGH-FIELD STRUCTURAL MR IMAGING OF MULTIPLE SCLEROSIS

The HF enables acquisition of high-resolution images, which along with high susceptibility produces an opportunity to probe the microstructure of brain tissues. Smaller voxels at HF reduces partial volume effect, whereas higher susceptibility increases T2* contrast between GM and WM. For example, GRE images acquired at 8.0 T from brain tissues of patients who have MS have shown higher sensitivity to demyelination lesions than seen at lower fields. The GRE and SE high-resolution images (100 μm in-plane resolution) of brain samples of newly deceased patients who had MS (see **Fig. 5**) at 8 T show the ability to visualize cortical microanatomy.[37] In these images, multilaminar structures have been revealed in the cortical gray matter (CGM) and at the same time cortical gray matter plaques are clearly seen. CGM plaques do not show up in routine clinical imaging at 1.5 T or even 3.0 T. Clearly, such work demonstrates that characteristics of MR images at high fields are relevant to the internal structure of CGM revealing them on 8.0 T images. The most prominent of these characteristics is the ability to acquire signal from smaller voxels. This property solely affects the number of excess protons in an ensemble of protons. Furthermore, equally high-resolution images acquired at lower fields using long acquisition time have not shown similar CGM plaques, leading one to conjecture that HF properties other than mere SNR must also play a role in enhancing the contrast to help visualize CGM plaques. Higher susceptibility and longer

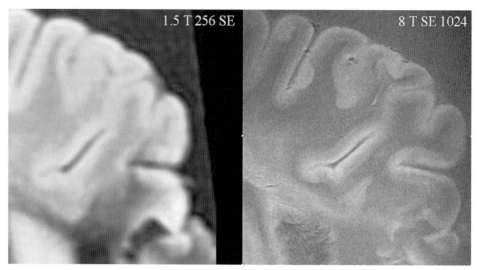

Fig. 5. Images acquired postmortem at 8.0 T from brain slices of a recently deceased patients who had MS. The GRE image on the right acquired with 100 μm in-plane resolution clearly shows CGM lesions. Compared to the image at 8.0 T on the right, the image on the left acquired at 1.5 T with voxels 10 times larger shows no clear sign of CGM lesions.

T1 values further contribute to contrast and SNR to reveal microstructures. As seen in **Fig. 5**, CGM plaques are visible on 8 T SE images with 1024 × 1024 matrix but they are not seen on 1.5 T images. Submillimeter resolutions achievable within clinically acceptable acquisition time enable 100 μm in-plane resolution capable of detecting CGM lesions with a contrast that easily lends itself to volumetric studies. Such high-resolution volumetric measurement offers a new tool for diagnosis and treatment of MS.

MR SPECTROSCOPY

Spectroscopy based on proton or other MR-detectable nuclei has been shown to be rich in information about many important metabolites. In normal human brain, MRS can detect N-acetylaspartate, choline-containing compounds, creatine/phosphocreatine, and lactate. Specialized editing techniques can even detect GABA, glutamate, glucose, and myoinositol. Despite the capability of MRS in detecting specific molecules, it has not yet been widely used in the clinical arena because of several factors. MRS at clinical field strength still suffers from low SNR and chemical shift dispersion (CSD). Furthermore, MRS is highly sensitive to B_0-homogeneity making higher-order shimming important for its acquisition. As static magnetic field increases, combination of SNR and CSD improves the sensitivity of MRS enabling acquisition of high-resolution in vivo spectra. Short TE MRS has been shown to be useful for detecting some metabolites invisible at long TE. Short TE spectra depend on high CSD, which makes it all

the more important to take full advantage of this feature of HF MRS to uncover signal from metabolites whose peaks overlap at low fields. Preliminary MRS work at 7.0 T has proved these capabilities by showing a large number of metabolites in the brain (**Fig. 6**).

Ability of HF to decouple some of the strongly coupled metabolites makes it a reliable tool to provide physiologic information about events at the cellular and molecular level. This fact is augmented by the large disparity between concentration of water (ie, 110 mol/L) used in imaging and metabolites at mmol/L and μmol/L detected in MRS. The five to eight orders of magnitude lower concentration of metabolites makes HF necessary for their reliable detection. The primary clinical sequences using images with 1-mm in-plane pixel

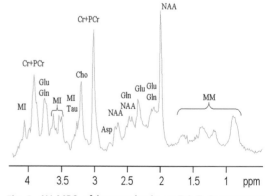

Fig. 6. 1H-MRS of human brain at 7.0 T. Parameters: STEAM, TE/TR = 15/3000, voxel volume = 3 cm³ NA: 256, location: parietal gray matter. (*Courtesy of Dr. Larry Wald, MGH NMR-Center, Boston, MA, USA.*)

dimensions and coupled to 5-mm slice thickness have been shown to lack sufficient SNR and CSD to offer a consistent quantification of major metabolite concentration in the human brain. Voxels of 1 mm^3 are possible for in vivo measurements at HF, which opens a whole new avenue in neuroscience research. Ability of generating high-resolution metabolite maps will address the difficult problem of voxel contamination and delineation of tissue boundaries. These features of HF MR imaging will improve specificity of findings by allowing reproducible measurement of the underlying molecular basis of tissue structure. In addition to MS, improvement offered by HF MRS could lead to a better understanding of many severe pathologic conditions, such as schizophrenia, autism, cancer, and stroke.

In MS, the capabilities offered by HF could shed light on the role of neurons and neuronal processes, because N-acetylasartate (NAA) resonance is readily detected in the brain. Accurate NAA values from WM will offer a specific marker of axonal integrity, which should allow a better assessment of the relationship between clinical manifestations of MS, demyelination, and axonal injury. Furthermore, combined improvements of SNR and CSD at 7.0 T could help quantify the possible reversibility of axonal injury and demyelination. In addition, HF ability of detection and identification of less abundant but important neural metabolites will contribute to better understanding the biochemical basis of functional impairment in MS. In other areas of neuroscience, the ability to remove coupling between spins will dramatically enhance detection of metabolites, such as glutamate and GABA, which are important regulators of CNS development[45,46] and have been used in the treatment of spasticity in MS.[47]

FUNCTIONAL MR IMAGING

fMR imaging, a noninvasive technique capable of detecting the brain response to an external stimulation, has experienced an explosive growth since its inception in 1990.[48] BOLD is the most widely used form of contrast in fMR imaging with the ability to provide functional information on the living brain.[5,48,49] There are many indications that medicine in general and MS in particular could greatly benefit from the potential of fMR imaging to unravel the basis of many diseases,[50,51] as demonstrated by BOLD fMR imaging studies conducted for the clinical assessment of MS. Research in various forms of fMR imaging holds great promise in sorting out diagnostic heterogeneity and treatment planning in MS, Alzheimer disease, Parkinson disease, brain tumors, and psychiatric disorders. fMR imaging at HF is capable of acquiring high-resolution functional maps of the brain regions (ie, approaching the submillimeter scale) (**Fig. 7**).[52,53] At present, although techniques such as PET, psychophysical measurements, and EEG are available to scientists, the ability to probe different areas of the brain by designing paradigms that target those areas will greatly advance the field. At HF, high-resolution fMR imaging could be used to assess the drug-induced signal changes in brain areas believed to be involved with generating a particular disorder. Taken together, the work of many investigators points to a new application of fMR imaging in monitoring the effect of drugs targeting specific brain structures.[54–58] Such use of fMR imaging lends itself more effectively to medical research.

The capabilities described previously will greatly help researchers in acquiring more precise functional maps with the ability to more exactly account for the underlying neuronal mechanism of those maps. The resolving power of submillimeter fMR imaging maps will provide an edge to researchers that could be incorporated subsequently into patient care. Furthermore, the HF will allow developmental work to improve our understanding of the nature of the fMR imaging signal and the underlying mechanisms of physiologic noise and the BOLD response.[55]

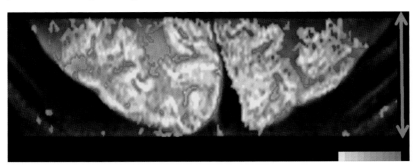

Fig. 7. Single shot SE-EPI fMR imaging acquired at 7.0 T with the following parameters: FOV: 2.5 × 12.8 cm^2, resolution: 0.5 × 0.5 × 3 mm^3, TR/TE: 2s/50 milliseconds, visual cortex, flashing checkerboard (5-minute scan). (*Courtesy of* Dr. Essa Yacoub, University of Minnesota.)

Functional imaging will also benefit from imaging at 7.0 T because magnetic susceptibility and consequently the BOLD effect will increase more than linearly with B_0. The high SNR of SE BOLD at 7.0 T will eliminate contributions of large draining veins to the signal, which will allow signal from microvascular capillary beds, directly over the site of neuronal activity, to be detected directly.[53] Such tools will enhance our ability to detect and precisely localize sites of functional abnormality in diseased brains, such as in individuals who have autism. Perfusion-based functional imaging will also benefit from the prolonged T1 at HF, which will enhance sensitivity in arterial spin-labeling studies. This imaging can provide quantitative measures of absolute cerebral blood flow, a more direct representation of neuronal activity than the BOLD signal.

SUMMARY

SNR is the highest award at HF. It is important to use this currency to enhance MR sensitivity and specificity in MS diagnostics or therapy. Although MR imaging is far more sensitive than CT for detecting MS lesions, the disease is still diagnosed clinically. The use of HF advantages to improve MR imaging specificity is helpful to take advantage of all MR imaging modalities. In MS, high SNR will enable plaques in many regions that are presently difficult to image, like posterior fossa, to be detected with higher sensitivity. Providing a sensitive marker for disease diagnosis, progression monitoring, and therapeutic efficacy is what HF MR imaging is expected to eventually offer in MS. MR imaging at field strengths of up to 3.0 T has yet not fulfilled that promise. Can higher fields help MR imaging fulfill its full potential? An affirmative answer to this question requires more refinement of the ancillary technologies, such as parallel imaging, and more thorough analysis of distinct aspects of HF beneficial to MS diagnosis and management.

REFERENCES

1. Bloch F. Nuclear induction. Phys Rev 1946;7:460–73.
2. Pourcell EM, Torrey HC, Pound RV. Resonance absorption by nuclear magnetic moments in a solid. Phys Rev 1946;69:37–8.
3. Lauterbur PC. Image formation by induced local interactions: example employing nuclear magnetic resoncance. Nature 1973;242:190–1.
4. Hoult DI, Lauterbur PC. The sensitivity of the zeumatographic experiment involving human samples. J Magn Reson 1979;34:425–33.
5. Ogawa S, Tank DW, Menon R, et al. Intrinsic signal changes accompanying sensory stimulation: functional brain mapping with magnetic resonance imaging. Proc Natl Acad Sci U S A 1992;89: 5951–5.
6. Hoult DI, Busby SJ, Gadian DG, et al. Observation of tissue metabolites using 31P nuclear magnetic resonance. Nature 1974;252:285–7.
7. Basser P. Inferring microstructural features and the physiological state of tissues from diffusion-weighted images. NMR Biomed 1995;8: 333–3344.
8. Christoforidis GA, Bourekas EC, Baujan M, et al. High resolution MRI of the deep brain vascular anatomy at 8 tesla: susceptibility-based enhancement of the venous structures. J Comput Assist Tomogr 1999;23:857–66.
9. Duewell S, Wolff SD, Wen H, et al. MR imaging contrast in human brain tissue: assessment and optimization at 4T. Radiology 1996;199:780–6.
10. Vetter J, Ries G, Reichert T. A 4-tesla superconducting whole-body magnet for MR imaging and spectroscopy. IEEE Trans Magn 1988;24:1285–7.
11. Barfuss H, Fischer H, Hentschel D, et al. Whole-body MR imaging and spectroscopy with a 4-T system. Radiology 1988;169:811–6.
12. Bomsdorf H, Helzel T, Kunz D, et al. Spectroscopy and imaging with a 4 tesla whole-body MR system. NMR Biomed 1988;1:151–6.
13. Ugurbil K, Adriany G, Andersen P, et al. Ultrahigh field magnetic resonance imaging and spectroscopy. Magn Reson Imaging 2003;21:1263–81.
14. Robitaille PM, Abduljalil AM, Kangarlu A, et al. Human magnetic resonance imaging at 8 T. NMR Biomed 1998;11:263–5.
15. Robitaille PM, Warner R, Jagadeesh J, et al. Design and assembly of an 8 tesla whole-body MR scanner. J Comput Assist Tomogr 1999;23:808–20.
16. Kangarlu A, Robitaille PML. Biological effects and implications in magnetic resonance imaging. Proceedings of International Society of Magnetic Resonance in Medicine 2000;12:321–59.
17. Kangarlu A, Burgess RE, Zhu H, et al. Cognitive, cardiac and physiological safety studies in ultra high field magnetic resonance imaging. Magn Reson Imaging 1999;17:1407–16.
18. Kangarlu A, Shellock FG. Aneurysm clips: evaluation of magnetic field interactions with an 8.0 T MR system. J Magn Reson Imaging 2000;12:107–11.
19. Budinger TF. Emerging nuclear magnetic resonance technologies. In: Magin RL, Liburdy RP, Persson B, editors. Biological effects and safety aspects of nuclear magnetic resonance imaging and spectroscopy. Annals of the New York Academy of Sciences. New York: New York Academy of Science; 1992. p. 1–18.
20. Keltner JR, Roos MS, Brakeman PR, et al. Magneto-hydrodynamics of blood flow. Magn Reson Med 1990;16:139–49.

21. Wright PJ, Mougin OE, Totman JJ, et al. Water proton T (1) measurements in brain tissue at 7, 3, and 1.5 T using IR-EPI, IR-TSE, and MPRAGE: results and optimization. MAGMA 2008;21:121–30.

22. Yacoub E, Duong TQ, Van De Moortele PF, et al. Spin-echo fMRI in humans using high spatial resolutions and high magnetic fields. Magn Reson Med 2003;49:655–64.

23. Vymazal J, Righini A, Brooks RA, et al. T1 and T2 in the brain of healthy subjects, patients with Parkinson disease, and patients with multiple system atrophy: relation to iron content. Radiology 1999; 211:489–95.

24. Liu F, Garland M, Duan Y, et al. Study of the development of fetal baboon brain using magnetic resonance imaging at 3 tesla. Neuroimage 2008;1(40): 148–59.

25. Robitaille PM, Abduljalil AM, Kangarlu A. Ultra high resolution imaging of the human head at 8 tesla: 2K × 2K for Y2K. J Comput Assist Tomogr 2000; 24:2–8.

26. McCoy MA, Ernst RR. Nuclear spin noise at room temperature. Chem Phys Lett 1989;159:587–93.

27. Hoult DI, Chen CN, Sank VJ. The field dependence of NMR imaging: II. arguments concerning an optimal field strength. Magn Reson Med 1986;3:730–46.

28. McDermott R, Lee S, ten Haken B, et al. Microtesla MRI with a superconducting quantum interference device. Proc Natl Acad Sci U S A 2004;101: 7857–61.

29. Wen H, Chesnick AS, Balaban RS. The design and test of a new volume coil for high field imaging. Magn Reson Med 1994;32:492–8.

30. Hoult DI, Richards RE. The signal-to-noise ratio of nuclear magnetic resonance experiment. J Magn Reson 1976;24:71–85.

31. Fatterpekar GM, Delman BN, Boonn WW, et al. MR microscopy of normal human brain. Magn Reson Imaging Clin N Am 2003;11:641–53.

32. Morris CM, Candy JM, Oakley AF, et al. Histochemical distribution of non-haem iron in the human brain. Acta Anat 1992;144:235–57.

33. Christoforidis GA, Kangarlu A, Abduljalil AM, et al. Susceptibility-based imaging of glioblastoma microvascularity at 8 T: correlation of MR imaging and postmortem pathology. AJNR Am J Neuroradiol 2004;25:756–60.

34. Duyn JH, van Gelderen P, Li TQ, et al. Free in PMC High-field MRI of brain cortical substructure based on signal phase. Proc Natl Acad Sci U S A 2007; 104:11796–801.

35. Chakeres DW, Kangarlu A, Abduljalil AM, et al. "High resolution UHFMRI of the human cerebral vasculature patterns". Proceedings of International Society of Magnetic Resonance in Medicine 2000;8:448.

36. Abduljalil AM, Schmalbrock P, Novak V, et al. Enhanced gray and white matter contrast of phase susceptibility-weighted images in ultra-high-field magnetic resonance imaging. J Magn Reson Imaging 2003;18:284–90.

37. Kangarlu A, Bourekas EC, Ray-Chaudhury A, et al. Free full text cerebral cortical lesions in multiple sclerosis detected by MR imaging at 8 tesla. AJNR Am J Neuroradiol 2007;28:262–6.

38. Kangarlu A, Baertlein BA, Lee R, et al. Dielectric resonance phenomena in ultra high field magnetic resonance imaging. J Comput Assist Tomogr 1999; 23:820–31.

39. Kangarlu A, Abduljalil AM, Robitaille PML. T1 and T2 weighted imaging at 8 tesla. J Comput Assist Tomogr 1999;23:875–8.

40. Pruessmann KP, Weiger M, Scheidegger MB, et al. SENSE: sensitivity encoding for fast MRI. Magn Reson Med 1999;42:952–62.

41. Sodickson DK, Manning WJ. Simultaneous acquisition of spatial harmonics (SMASH): fast imaging with radiofrequency coil arrays. Magn Reson Med 1997;38:591–603.

42. Jackson GD, Connelly A, Duncan JS, et al. Detection of hippocampal pathology in intractable partial epilepsy: increased sensitivity with quantitative magnetic resonance T2 relaxometry. Neurology 1993;43:1793–9.

43. Van Paesschen W, Revesz T, Duncan JS, et al. Quantitative neuropathology and quantitative magnetic resonance imaging of the hippocampus in temporal lobe epilepsy. Ann Neurol 1997;42: 756–66.

44. Van Paesschen W, Connelly A, Johnson CL, et al. The amygdala and intractable temporal lobe epilepsy: a quantitative magnetic resonance imaging study. Neurology 1996;47:1021–31, Erratum in: Neurology 1997;48:1751.

45. Bhagwagar Z, Wylezinska M, Taylor M, et al. Increased brain GABA concentrations following acute administration of a selective serotonin reuptake inhibitor. Am J Psychiatry 2004;161: 368–70.

46. Rothman DL, Sibson NR, Hyder F, et al. In vivo nuclear magnetic resonance spectroscopy studies of the relationship between the glutamate-glutamine neurotransmitter cycle and functional neuroenergetics. Philosophical Transactions of the Royal Society of London 1999;354:1165–77.

47. Rudick RA, Breton D, Krall RL. The GABA-agonist progabide for spasticity in multiple sclerosis 1. Arch Neurol 1987;44:1033–6.

48. Ogawa S, Lee TM, Nayak AS, et al. Oxygenation-sensitive contrast in magnetic resonance image of rodent brain at high magnetic fields. Magn Reson Med 1990;14:68–78.

49. Kim SG, Ugurbil K. High-resolution functional magnetic resonance imaging of the animal brain. Methods 2003;30:28–41.

50. Meltzer HY, McGurk SR. The effects of cloza-pine, risperidone, and olanzapine on cognitive function in schizophrenia. Schizophr Bull 1999; 25:233–55.

51. Sadek JR, Hammeke TA. Functional neuroimaging in neurology and psychiatry. CNS Spectr 2002;7: 286–90. 295–9.

52. Logothetis N, Merkle H, Augath M, et al. Ultra high-resolution fMRI in monkeys with implanted RF coils. Neuron 2002;35:227–42.

53. Yacoub E, Shmuel A, Pfeuffer J, et al. Imaging brain function in humans at 7 tesla. Magn Reson Med 2001;45:588–94.

54. Bloom AS, Hoffmann RG, Fuller SA, et al. Determination of drug-induced changes in functional MRI signal using a pharmacokinetic model. Hum Brain Mapp 1999;8:235–44.

55. Stein EA, Pankiewicz J, Harsch HH, et al. Nicotine-induced limbic cortical activation in the human brain: a functional MRI study. Am J Psychiatry 1998;155:1009–15.

56. Loubinoux I, Boulanouar K, Ranjeva JP, et al. Cerebral functional magnetic resonance imaging activation modulated by a single dose of the monoamine neurotransmission enhancers fluoxetine and fenozo-lone during hand sensorimotor tasks. J Cereb Blood Flow Metab 1999;19:1365–75.

57. Suzuki M, Zhou SY, Takahashi T, et al. Differential contributions of prefrontal and temporolimbic pathology to mechanisms of psychosis. Brain 2005;128:2109–22.

58. Wansapura JP, Holland SK, Dunn RS, et al. NMR relaxation times in the human brain at 3.0 tesla. J Magn Reson Imaging 1999;9:531–8.

Index

Neuroimag Clin N Am 19 (2009) 129–132
doi:10.1016/S1052-5149(08)00126-3
1052-5149/08/$ – see front matter © 2008 Elsevier Inc. All rights reserved.

neuroimaging.theclinics.com

Moving?

Make sure your subscription moves with you!

To notify us of your new address, find your **Clinics Account Number** (located on your mailing label above your name), and contact customer service at:

E-mail: elspcs@elsevier.com

800-654-2452 (subscribers in the U.S. & Canada)
314-453-7041 (subscribers outside of the U.S. & Canada)

Fax number: 314-523-5170

Elsevier Periodicals Customer Service
11830 Westline Industrial Drive
St. Louis, MO 63146

*To ensure uninterrupted delivery of your subscription, please notify us at least 4 weeks in advance of move.